Myths & Facts
about lung cancer

What you need to know

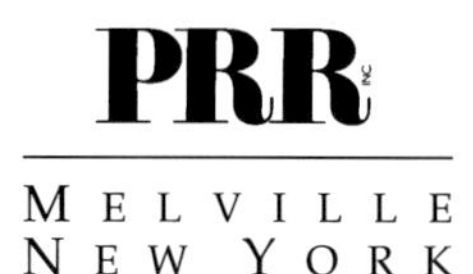

Publishers of ONCOLOGY
Oncology News International
Primary Care & Cancer
Managed Care & Cancer
In Touch: The Good Health Guide to Cancer
     Prevention and Treatment
Cancer Management: A Multidisciplinary Approach
Myths and Fact Series

PRR
M E L V I L L E
N E W   Y O R K

Myths & Facts
about lung cancer

What you need to know

JOHN C. RUCKDESCHEL, MD
Professor of Medicine and Director
H. Lee Moffitt Cancer Center
and Research Institute at the
University of South Florida
Tampa, Florida

Jacket artwork and text illustrations by Ron Futral.

About the Author

John C. Ruckdeschel, MD, serves as the Center Director and Chief Executive Officer of the H. Lee Moffitt Cancer Center and Research Institute, a National Cancer Institute-designated cancer center. He is Professor of Medicine at the University of South Florida College of Medicine and Professor in the Department of Community and Family Health at the University of South Florida College of Public Health. Dr. Ruckdeschel received a BSc degree in Biology from Rennselaer Polytechnic Institute and his MD degree from Albany Medical College, Albany, New York. He trained at Johns Hopkins, Harvard, and the National Cancer Institute.

Prior to joining the Moffitt Cancer Center, he was Director of the Joint Center for Cancer and Blood Disorders, as well as the division head of Medical Oncology at Albany Medical College. Dr. Ruckdeschel is both a nationally and internationally recognized physician and leader in the field of medical oncology, particularly in the area of lung cancer. He is a Fellow of the American College of Chest Physicians, co-editor of the "Textbook of Thoracic Oncology," I & II editions, and was appointed by the governor as a member of the Florida Cancer Control and Research Advisory Committee.

Dr. Ruckdeschel's curriculum vitae is highlighted by an impressive and lengthy list of publications. In addition, he is a sought-after site reviewer for cancer-related programs and research activities.

Contents

Introduction 11

What Is Lung Cancer? 13
  The Four Types of Lung Cancers 15

What Causes Lung Cancer? 16
  The First Mutation 16
  The Second Mutation 17
  Smoking and Lung Cancer 17
    Former Smokers and Lung Cancer 18
    Nonsmokers and Lung Cancer 19
    Environmental Smoke 20

What Are the Symptoms of Lung Cancer? 21
  Symptoms of Local Lung Cancer 21
  Symptoms of Regional (Locally Advanced) Lung Cancer 22
  Symptoms of Distant (Widespread) Lung Cancer 26

How Is Lung Cancer Diagnosed? 28
  The Physical Examination 30
  Diagnostic Tests 31
    Tests for Presumed Local or Regional Disease 31
    Tests for Presumed Distant (Widespread) Disease 35

Lung Cancer Staging—
Its Definition and Significance 36
  T Stage 36
  N Stage 38
  M Stage 40
  Stages 1 Through 4 40
    Stage 1 Disease 42
    Stage 2 Disease 42
    Stage 3 Disease 42
    Stage 4 Disease 42

Continued on the following page

Contents *continued*

Non-Small-Cell Lung Cancer 43
Treating Stage 1 Non-Small-Cell Lung Cancer 43
Treating Stage 2 Non-Small-Cell Lung Cancer 45
Treating Stage 3 Non-Small-Cell Lung Cancer 46
Treating Stage 4 Non-Small-Cell Lung Cancer 47
Chemotherapy for Non-Small-Cell Lung Cancer 48
New Drugs 49

Small-Cell Lung Cancer 51
Two Presentations of Small-Cell Lung Cancer:
Limited and Extensive 51
Limited Small-Cell Lung Cancer 51
Extensive Small-Cell Lung Cancer 52
Treating Small-Cell Lung Cancer 52
Treating Limited Small-Cell Lung Cancer 52
Treating Extensive Small-Cell Lung Cancer 54
Nuances of Small-Cell Lung Cancer 54
Brain Metastases 55
Carcinoid and Atypical Carcinoid Tumors 56
Vaccine and Gene Therapies for Small-Cell Lung Cancer 57

The Follow-Up Treatment of Lung Cancer 58
The Follow-Up Examination 58
The Patient in Remission 59
The Problem of "Second Primary" Cancers 60
Diagnosis of a Second Primary Cancer 61

How Can Lung Cancer Be Prevented? 62
Primary Prevention 62
Adolescent Smoking 62
Adult Smoking 63
Secondary Prevention 64
Antioxidants and Natural Vitamins 64

How to Cope With Lung Cancer 66
Second Opinions 66
Family Involvement 67
Dealing With Pain 67
Hair Loss 68
Releasing the Guilt 68
Managing Breathing Problems 69
Hospices 70
Support Groups 70

**Appendix: Support Groups and
Resources for Lung Cancer Patients** 72

Glossary 73

Introduction

LUNG CANCER!

In the early 1900s, before the epidemic of cigarette smoking began in earnest, lung *cancer* was a rare disease. It has now become one of the greatest public health scourges ever to befall mankind. A diagnosis of lung cancer brings on many emotions, chief among them, fear. This fear is often accompanied by a feeling of guilt at having caused this cancer by continued cigarette smoking, despite the knowledge that it was harmful.

Lung cancer patients and their families receive copious amounts of unsolicited advice that can vary from helpful to nonsensical. However, with lung cancer, more than almost any other cancer, the message most often transmitted by friends, physicians, and other healthcare workers is pessimism. Therapeutic nihilism, or a hesitancy to trust and utilize lung cancer treatments, has long characterized the medical profession's approach to lung cancer. Unfortunately, the world of cancer specialists has not been far behind in its pessimism about the treatment of this disease. Those nostrums and "old wives tales" passed on by well-meaning, but uninformed, acquaintances and medical professionals make it difficult for lung cancer patients to receive and interpret the information they need to make proper decisions about their treatment options.

We, as cancer specialists, realize that patients with lung cancer are often asked to make prompt treatment decisions during a period of intense personal and familial crises. This handbook was designed to provide you with the information you will need to work with your physician to identify what can and cannot be done to help treat your disease. It was also designed to help you weigh the individual risks and benefits of the various diagnostic and treatment options available to you. This booklet is

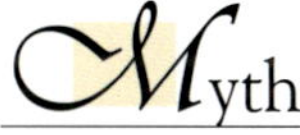

Myth

All lung cancers are fatal.

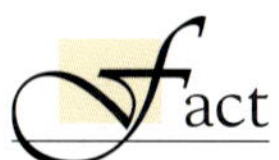

Fact

No, they're not. Significant progress has been made in multiple areas of treatment, including surgery, radiation therapy, **chemotherapy**, and **combined modality** therapy.

not a comprehensive guide to treatment options—
They are changing every day. It will, however, help
you understand the fundamental issues related to
the development of lung cancer, from its propensity
to spread, to its responsiveness to various forms of
treatment. Armed with this information, you will
then be able to make rational, thoughtful decisions
about your treatment.

Unfortunately, myths and misconceptions about
lung cancer are still very common, the greatest
among them being that surgery is the only effective
treatment. It is imperative that you as a patient or
family member recognize that this information is
false, and that its continued "blind" acceptance by
many in the medical profession and lay communities costs people years of useful life.

In this book, we will identify the most common
myths about lung cancer and try to give you the
facts about this disease. We consider this handbook
one that can be read at home, at work, or in a physician's office. It can be read from beginning to end,
or you can turn directly to a specific topic in which
you are interested. Throughout this booklet, you
will also find bold, italicized words, which are defined more fully in the glossary on page 73. In addition, you will find quotes from former lung cancer
patients, who, in their own words, describe their
feelings during and after treatment. We remain
perpetually indebted to these individuals for their
openness and willingness to help others affected by
this disease.

২

What Is Lung Cancer?

The lung is a complex organ. Most of us associate the lung with breathing. We fail to recognize that the lung plays the following significant roles. The lung:

- localizes and repels various infectious organisms,
- helps maintain water balance, and
- produces a number of hormones.

The cells that make up the lining of your lungs look very much like the inside lining of your cheek. The cellular structure of the lung tissues is far more complex, however. The lung (**Figure 1**) consists of three different zones:

1) The cells that line the *trachea* (*windpipe*) and the first portion of the *large airways* (*bronchi*) are flat (squamoid). These cells serve as a protective layer against various inhaled substances.

2) The more central zones of the lung, often referred to as the *secretory zone*, are lined with a series of cells that produce a very thin watery mucus. Tiny hairs on these *ciliated cells* constantly move this thin mucus—in which our various inhaled particles are trapped—from the outer portions of the lung, up through the windpipe, and ultimately to the mouth, where we swallow them.

3) The farthest portions of the lung consist of literally millions of tiny air sacs, called *alveoli*. In the alveoli, the exchange of oxygen and carbon dioxide (the process of breathing) takes place. Here too, the process of controlling the body's water balance via evaporation occurs.

Each of these three areas, or zones, of the lung is affected differently by the toxic products in cigarette smoke. As we will discuss later, some lung cancers can spontaneously arise without a history of smoking. However, the vast majority of lung cancers results from previous heavy, sustained smoking.

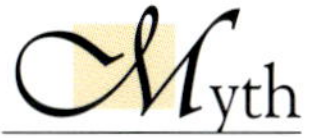

Myth

All lung cancers are the same.

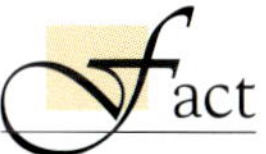

Fact

No, they're not. A cascade of mutations leads to varying patterns of cancer growth (small-cell, non-small-cell), varying rates of cancer growth, varying abilities to spread, and varying abilities to resist therapy.

FIGURE I

Anatomy of the lungs—This illustration shows the lungs, bronchi, and adjacent anatomy in the chest cavity.

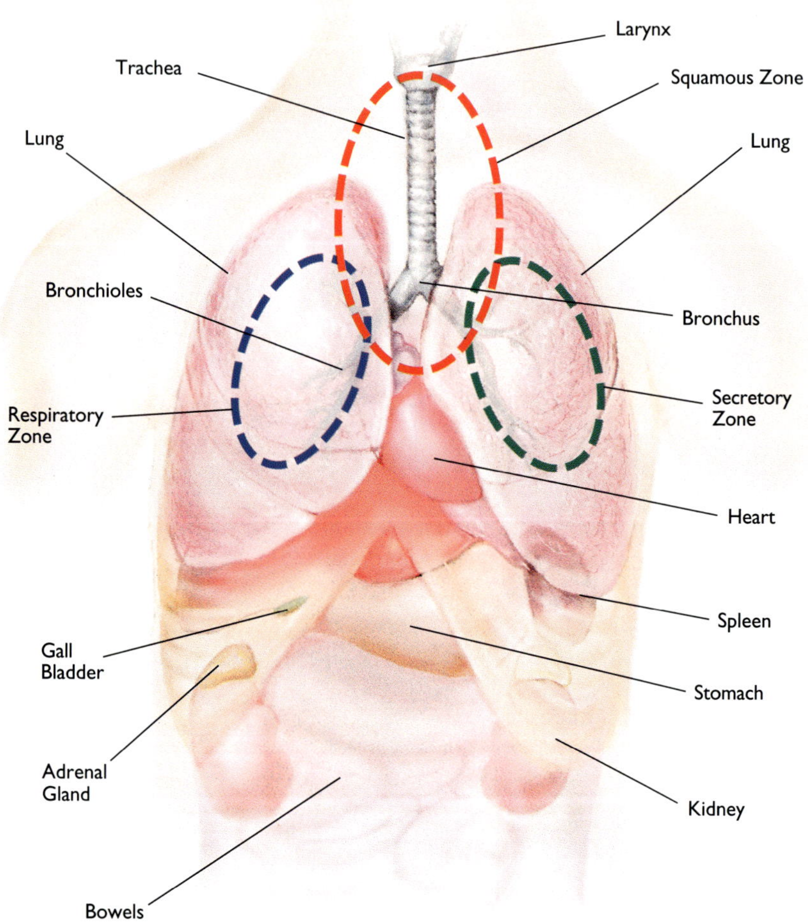

One of the first effects of cigarette smoke on the airways is the destruction of the ciliated cells that help the body move inhaled particles, including smoke particles, out of the body. Eventually, inflammation of the smaller airways **(bronchitis)** and destruction and coalescence of the tiny air sacs occur **(emphysema)**. The process of sustaining the normal lining of the airway and repairing the damage caused by smoking is one that is quite tightly controlled in the healthy lung.

"Ask all the questions you can. There's a lot of information out there just for the taking."

THE FOUR TYPES OF LUNG CANCERS

Whenever cancer specialists think about lung cancer, or any cancer for that matter, we need to answer two fundamental questions in order to plan treatment: "What type of cancer does the patient have?" and "Where is the patient's cancer?"

There are four types of lung cancers, none of which are alike:

• *small-cell lung cancers* are cancers that arise from the hormonal cells in the lung, and

• *non-small-cell lung cancers*, which include:

—*squamous-cell cancers*, which arise in the larger airways;

—*adenocarcinomas* (including large-cell carcinomas), which occur in the secretory portion of the lung; and

—*bronchoalveolar carcinomas*, which arise in the cells that make up the small air sacs, or alveoli.

Each of these cancers retains some of the characteristics of the zone of the lung in which they arose, thereby behaving somewhat differently than the other forms of lung cancer. For convenience sake, we will break these four lung cancers into two major categories: small-cell lung cancers, which arise from the hormonal cells in the lungs, and all other forms of lung cancer, which we will refer to as non-small-cell lung cancers. As we will see, a correct diagnosis of the type of lung cancer, and more importantly, an understanding of the specific cancer's spread site(s), are key to determining a patient's therapy. These two key factors will also determine the likely outcome of the selected therapy.

What Causes Lung Cancer?

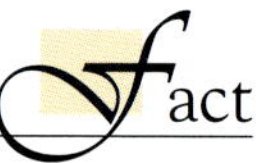

Myth

Smoking cessation offers little benefit to lowering lung cancer risk in an individual who has smoked for most of his or her life.

Fact

Smoking cessation will definitely reduce an individual's risk of death from lung cancer. The risk of developing lung cancer persists for more than a decade after an individual stops smoking, but is reduced with time, and after 10 years, is about half that of a continuing smoker.

When an individual cell in the lining of the lung becomes **malignant** (either from cigarette smoking or other factors we will touch on later), the body is unable to stop the cell's cancerous growth. This leads to a process of uncontrolled growth called **metastasis**. The events leading up to this malignant transformation represent a series of molecular changes that occur in an individual lung cell. **Figure 2** illustrates the progression of cancer from a normal lung **epithelium** (a tissue layer that lines the internal surfaces) to **hyperplasia** (an abnormal multiplication of cells) through the stages of **dysplasia** (an abnormal growth of cells), and finally, to cancer. After the process of malignant growth has culminated in a cancer, the process of mutation does not, unfortunately, stop. Among the many mutations that can occur after a cell becomes malignant, two are specifically dangerous:

THE FIRST MUTATION

The first mutation is the ability of a cancer cell to leave its original site and spread, or metastasize, to other areas of the body. When cancer cells arise in the lung and these cancer cells spread elsewhere in the body (eg, to the bone, liver, or brain), a patient is said to have lung cancer metastatic to these various parts of the body. This lung cancer patient will not be described, per se, as having cancer of the bone, liver, or brain. Furthermore, if this lung cancer patient's cancer has spread to the **lymph nodes/glands**, bones, or liver, he or she will need to understand the process of lung cancer, not lymph node cancer, bone cancer, or liver cancer. This is a common source of confusion for patients and their families.

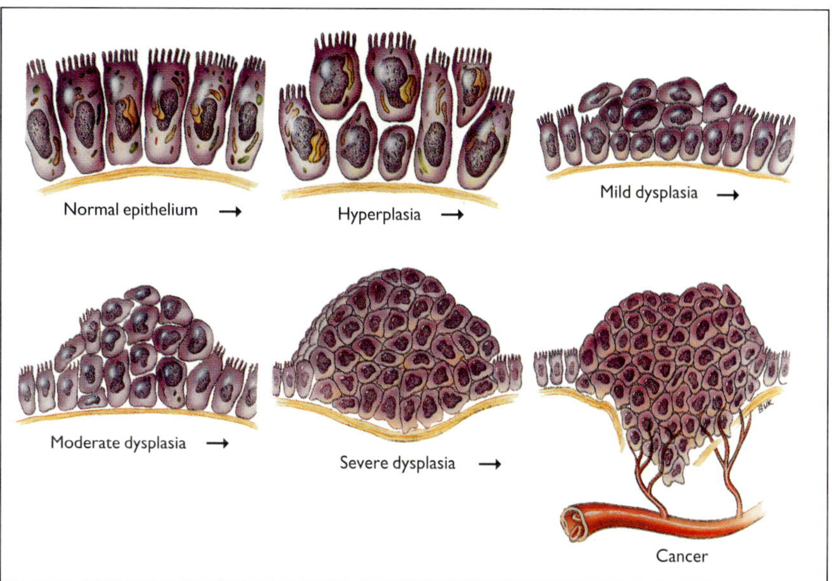

FIGURE 2

Progression to cancer—The process leading from the normal epithelium to cancer involves multiple steps, including progression from the normal epithelium to hyperplasia, and through the stages of dysplasia to cancer.

THE SECOND MUTATION

The second mutation is the lung cancer cell's learned ability to resist therapy. Although this can happen in many ways, it is usually caused by the cancer cell's ability to repair any therapy-induced "damage" faster than the normal cells of the body repair this damage, thereby making the delivery of effective doses of therapy too toxic for normal cells. When this happens, a cancer is said to be **resistant**, or **refractory**, to therapy.

SMOKING AND LUNG CANCER

There is little question that the toxic chemicals in cigarette smoke are the cause of the vast majority of lung cancers. However, a whole series of misunderstandings about the relationship between smoking and lung cancer still exist.

All of us have heard about the chronic smoker who refuses, or is unable, to stop smoking. Efforts

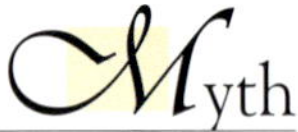

Most heavy smokers will develop lung cancer.

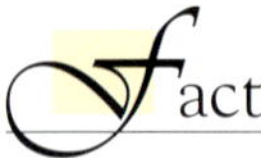

Most smokers will not develop lung cancer; some non-smokers will develop lung cancer.

made by family and friends to help this individual stop smoking are countered with stories about "Uncle Charlie," who is 80 years old and has smoked his entire life. Uncle Charlie is, however, an important illustration in the link between smoking and cancer.

Physicians define a significant smoker as someone who has at least "20-pack-years" of smoking history. This would equate to 1 pack per day for 20 years, 2 packs per day for 10 years, etc. A significant smoker only has a 10% to 15% chance, <u>at most</u>, of developing lung cancer. This means that 85% to 90% of heavy smokers will not develop lung cancer. This does not mean that they will not become ill and die prematurely; they most certainly will. However, they will die of emphysema, *chronic obstructive pulmonary disease (COPD)*, *peripheral vascular disease*, and *accelerated coronary artery disease*, instead of lung cancer. This strongly suggests that there is a genetic basis for deciphering which heavy smokers will develop lung cancer, and which will develop cardiopulmonary disorders. Unfortunately, although this gene is being actively pursued, it has not yet been identified.

Former Smokers and Lung Cancer: The most common presentation seen today is the patient who has stopped smoking anywhere from 1 to 10 years earlier, and who goes on to develop lung cancer anyway. This patient is often frustrated at having gone through the effort of smoking cessation only to find that he or she still developed cancer. However, it is important to understand that more than 10 years may pass before the transformation of a normal cell to a malignant cell presents as cancer. Consequently, the risk of developing lung cancer persists for over a decade after an individual stops smoking. **Table 1** depicts the number of cancer deaths attributable to smoking.

According to the National Cancer Institute, cessation of smoking will definitively reduce the risk of death from lung cancer. After 10 years of smoking cessation, the risk of lung cancer death among former smokers is about 50% the risk of continuing smokers. Those who reduce their daily usage and those who smoke filtered, low-tar cigarettes will gain some benefit; although their risk of developing lung cancer is still much higher than a nonsmoker's risk.

Nonsmokers and Lung Cancer: If there were no smoking-related cancers, lung cancer would be a rare disease indeed. But what about those people who develop lung cancer, but have never had heavy exposure to cigarette smoke? This group represents those patients in whom a *"spontaneous cancer"* develops. Oftentimes, these spontaneous cancers occur in younger women who develop a specific kind of lung cancer, called bronchoalveolar carcinoma.

TABLE I

1994 US CANCER DEATHS ATTRIBUTED TO CIGARETTE SMOKING

	1994 Cancer Deaths Expected	Smoking Attributable Risk %	Estimated Deaths Due To Smoking
MALES			
Oral	5,150	90.0	4,635
Esophagus	7,800	76.7	5,983
Pancreas	12,400	25.6	3,174
Larynx	3,000	79.3	2,379
Lung	94,000	89.2	83,848
Bladder	7,000	43.1	3,017
Kidney	6,800	44.6	3,033
Total Male Cancer Deaths Expected	**283,000**		**106,069 (37.5%)**
FEMALES			
Oral	2,775	58.5	1,624
Esophagus	2,600	71.6	1,862
Pancreas	13,500	31.2	4,212
Larynx	800	86.9	695
Lung	59,000	78.5	46,315
Cervix	4,600	30.8	1,417
Bladder	3,600	34.3	1,235
Kidney	4,500	15.3	689
Total Female Cancer Deaths Expected	**255,000**		**58,049 (22.8%)**
Total male and female cancer deaths expected in 1994			538,000
Total excess deaths attributed to cigarette smoking			164,118
Percentage attributed to cigarette smoking			30.5%

Source: The National Cancer Institute

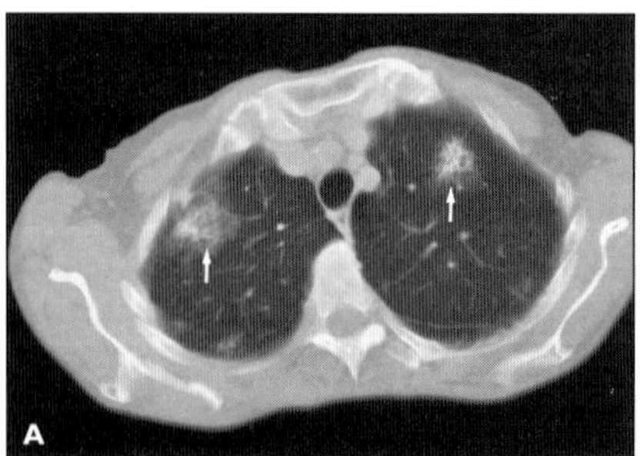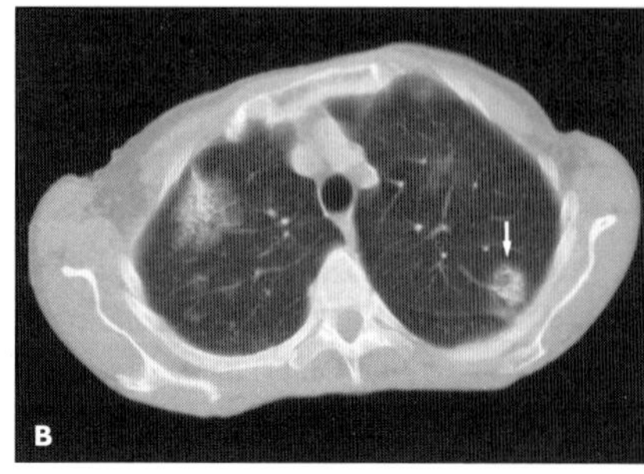

FIGURES 3A & B

*An example of multicentric bronchoalveolar carcinoma. Two CT slices obtained through the lung **apices** of the same patient. Irregular densities can be seen in both lungs. (A) The left mass yielded a diagnosis of bronchoalveolar cell carcinoma on biopsy. (B) Two days later, the right mass (white arrow) yielded the same diagnosis on biopsy.*

Figures 3(A) and **3(B)** depict a CT scan showing **multicentric** bronchoalveolar carcinoma. Unfortunately, it is not yet clear why these cancers are arising in this population of patients.

Environmental Smoke: There has been enormous interest in the problem of **environmental smoke** over the last several years. The data seem reasonably conclusive that significant environmental exposure over time can lead to an increased risk of lung cancer—even in those who are nonsmokers. The greatest risk, however, appears to be children who are chronically exposed to heavy smoke in their parents' home, and to employees who are in a closed working environment with constant exposure to cigarette smoke. Nonetheless, the full extent of the risk, while positively increased, is not yet clear.

Contrary to widespread belief, occasional exposure to casual cigarette smoke in a restaurant or public place will not cause lung cancer. There are, however, a number of **occupational** and **environmental exposures** that may enhance the risk of developing lung cancer. Asbestos, several different chronic dust exposures, and radon exposure all demonstrate a **synergistic effect**, leading to an increased rate of lung cancer.

What Are the Symptoms of Lung Cancer?

The cancer specialist's first goal is to find the cancer before it causes any symptoms. However, if that is not possible, it is certainly far superior to detect the cancer when there are only symptoms of *regional* (or *locally advanced*) *disease*, rather than symptoms of *distant* (or *widespread*) *disease*.

The symptoms of lung cancer **(Table 2)** may help identify whether the disease is *local*, regional, or distant.

SYMPTOMS OF LOCAL LUNG CANCER

Far and away, the most common symptom of a *primary tumor* is a cough. The *tumor* takes up space in the lungs and causes an irritation that an individual senses and tries to cough up. Because the vast majority of lung cancer patients are cigarette smokers, they often delude themselves into thinking their cough is merely an extension of their previous *"smoker's cough."* A smoker's cough may not yet herald the development of cancer, but it is abnormal. Consequently, a smoker who already has a smoker's cough needs to be particularly sensitive to a change in the pattern of that cough.

If the primary tumor erodes into a blood vessel in the airway, it can also cause bleeding into the airway, which is then coughed up and results in a noticeable spotting of the phlegm. This process is called *hemoptysis*.

The most prevalent presenting sign of localized lung cancer, however, is *pneumonia* in an adult that fails to resolve. If a tumor blocks an airway by either pressing on it from the outside, or by plugging

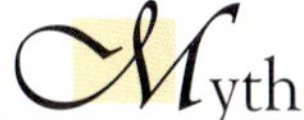

If I pay attention to the "early warning signs" of lung cancer (cough, chest discomfort, or coughing up blood), I will be able to diagnose it early enough to allow curative treatment.

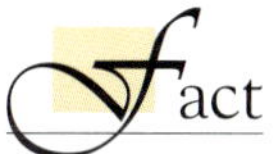

By the time an individual presents with any of the "warning signs" of lung cancer, the cancer is, unfortunately, already at a late stage. Lung cancer is one of the most notoriously difficult cancers to diagnose early.

it up by growth within the airway itself, an infection will develop beyond the obstructed area. This results in pneumonia and its traditional signs, including cough, the production of **purulent** sputum, and fever. Any adult who develops pneumonia should have a follow-up chest **x-ray** several weeks later; if the infiltrates have not cleared, a work-up for lung cancer should immediately ensue.

Many individuals will also have an obstruction and infection in their lung without being fully aware of it. The presentation of such an "asymptomatic" pneumonia in an adult smoker is, unfortunately, particularly ominous.

SYMPTOMS OF REGIONAL (LOCALLY ADVANCED) LUNG CANCER

The inside of the chest is a very complex place. Three fourths of the area surrounding the lung itself is what we call the chest wall. It is made up of a thin inner lining **(parietal pleura)**, fat, muscle, ribs, and skin in varying proportions. When a tumor invades any of these areas, it will cause pain. Therefore, the most common sign of regional spread of lung cancer within the chest is chest wall pain.

TABLE 2
COMMON SYMPTOMS OF LUNG CANCER

Local Lung Cancer	*Regional Lung Cancer*	*Distant Lung Cancer*
Cough	Chest wall pain	Relentless headache
Hemoptysis (blood in phlegm)	Hoarseness	Tension headache
Pneumonia (cough, purulent sputum, fever)	Distended neck veins	Blurred vision
	Arm pain/weakness	Confusion
	Shortness of breath	Seizures
	Facial/neck swelling	Rib discomfort
		Back/leg pain
		Weakness in legs
		Poor bowel/bladder control
		Fatigue
		Uncontrollable weight loss
		Paralysis

The above symptoms may present with either local, regional, or distant lung cancer.

A unique subset of the chest wall involves the very top—or *apex*—of the lung. In this area, the nerves that control the arm, both its movement and sensation, run from the lower portion of the neck, across the space at the top of the lung, and down the arm. Consequently, a tumor invading this area will often present with signs of pain and then weakness in the arm on the affected side. This so-called *Pancoast tumor*, or *superior sulcus tumor*, is a type of lung cancer that often masquerades as shoulder pain. The pain of a Pancoast tumor is often severe enough to require analgesics and narcotics. Oftentimes, a physician will refer a patient presenting with arm pain to an orthopedic surgeon or neurologist, thereby losing precious time in diagnosing a lung cancer. **Figure 4** depicts a Pancoast tumor.

Approximately one fourth of the lung's surface abuts what we call the **mediastinum**. This term, meaning "the middle of the chest," is a catch-all term for a space that encloses a number of vital

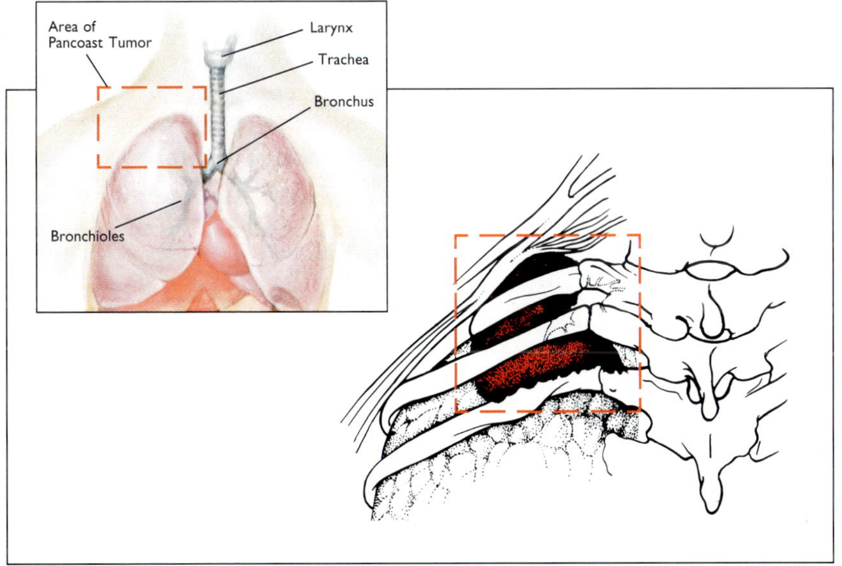

FIGURE 4
The red structure indicates a Pancoast tumor. The inset indicates the location of the tumor.

"I never paid attention to having regular check-ups. Now I know how necessary they are."

organs. The mediastinum exists directly behind the breastbone, and, in lay terms, is known as the solar plexus. The main airways, or bronchi, branch through the mediastinum. The esophagus, or swallowing tube, moves through this space directly behind the windpipe. The heart and all of its major blood vessels also occupy the mediastinum, as do several vital nerves. When cancer spreads into the mediastinum, the following symptoms may occur:

Hoarseness is one of the most common symptoms related to a regional spread of lung cancer. It is a fluke of embryology that the recurrent laryngeal nerve that controls our left vocal cord passes from the neck down into the chest, wraps around the main blood vessel coming from the heart, and goes back up the voice box to control the left vocal cord. Therefore, a tumor that has spread into the mediastinum's left side can press on this nerve, causing progressive hoarseness that is not accompanied by the usual sore throat or signs of an upper respiratory infection.

On the other side of the chest, a major vein, called the **superior vena cava,** drains all of the blood from the upper extremities and the head into the circulatory system. If a tumor invades the mediastinum's right side, it can compress this vein almost as if a tourniquet were being slowly applied. Initially, it may begin as distended veins in the neck, but eventually, significant swelling of the neck and face will occur. This is a true medical emergency and needs to be diagnosed promptly.

Ultimately, nearly all patients with locally advanced, or regional, lung cancer will also present with some degree of shortness of breath. Normal tissue fluids produced by the lung and heart muscles drain through the lymph nodes in the middle of the chest **(Figure 5)**. If these glands become blocked by a tumor, fluid can build up around the heart **(pericardial effusion)** or in the space between the lung and the inside of the chest wall **(pleural effusion)**. Patients with either of these conditions will present

FIGURE 5

Lymph nodes of the lungs—this illustration shows the location of two types of lymph nodes of the lungs and bronchial tubes; and the yellow arrows indicate the routes of lymph fluid drainage.

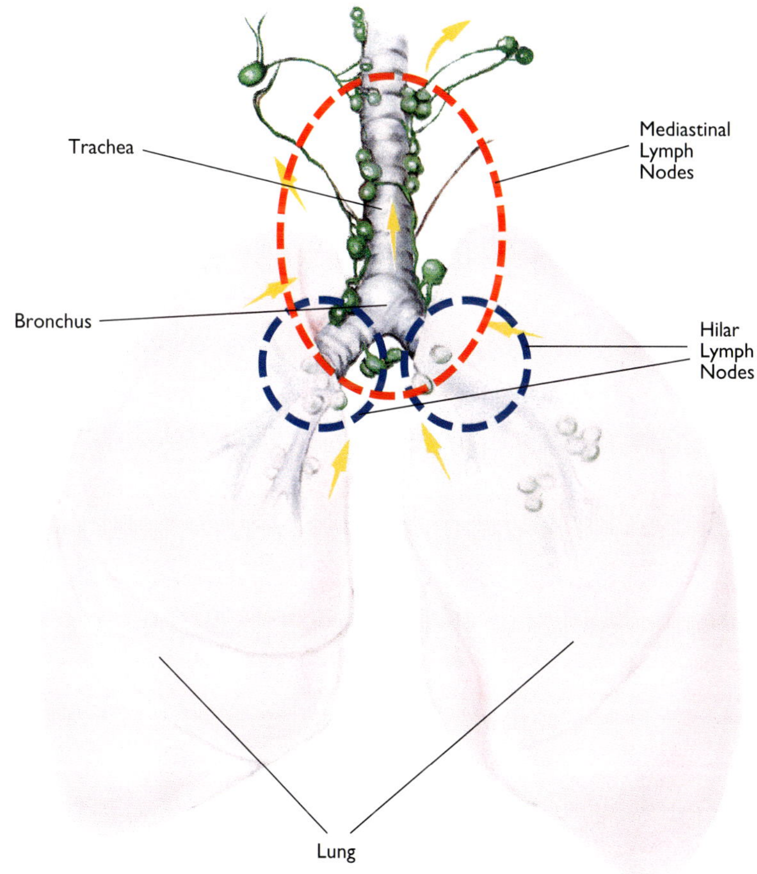

with shortness of breath. However, because many patients will also have some degree of chronic pulmonary disease from their smoking, this distinction may be difficult to decipher. Additionally, at some point, the amount of lung taken up by the tumor will cause the amount of remaining normal lung to fall below a level that is appropriate for comfortable breathing. Initially, this discomfort will occur with exercise, but eventually, it will occur at rest, as well.

All of the above symptoms imply regionally **advanced disease**. Regrettably, they portend a much poorer prognosis.

SYMPTOMS OF DISTANT (WIDESPREAD) LUNG CANCER

Because lung cancer tends to spread relatively early in its course, symptoms related to distant spread are often the very first sign a patient and his or her physician will notice. If cancer spreads to the brain, it may cause a continuous, relentless headache and some blurring of vision. As it worsens, confusion, and potentially, seizures, may follow. The nature of the headache may not be different than the traditional tension headache, so most people discount it. The blurring of vision usually presents as trouble reading a newspaper or watching television. Because most patients with lung cancer are older, they usually ascribe this to a need to change their eyeglass prescription. The key point is to watch for a change in previous patterns. Signs of confusion and change in visual acuity can be very subtle in the early stages.

When cancer spreads to the bone, it will cause destruction of the bone. Eventually, when sufficient bone is destroyed, pain will occur. If enough of the hard, outer shell of a bone **(cortex)** is destroyed, the bone may become structurally unstable. If this occurs in a rib, it may cause discomfort; but if it happens in one of the long bones that support the body, such as the thigh bone **(femur)**, or the main bone of

the upper arm *(humerus)*, the bone may even frac-
ture during routine activities.

Finally, and most ominously, the cancer may
invade the spine. An invasion into the spine will
cause pain in the vast majority of patients. A major
concern, however, is that the cancer will spread
further to the *spinal cord*, which is encased within
the spine itself. This would first present as back
pain, followed slowly by pain running down the
legs, weakness in the legs, trouble controlling the
bowel and bladder, and eventually, paralysis below
the point of compression. Back pain in a heavy
smoker should always be carefully evaluated.

However, the most common symptoms of distant, or widespread, disease are fatigue and weight
loss. Patients with active and distant cancer invari-
ably have unexplained weight loss. This is preceded
by a loss of appetite, and in time, no amount of
encouragement to eat will result in weight gain.

How Is Lung Cancer Diagnosed?

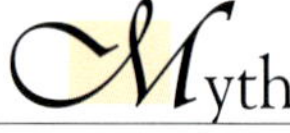

Myth

If only someone had taken a chest x-ray a few months ago, I could have found this cancer early, and not been in this predicament.

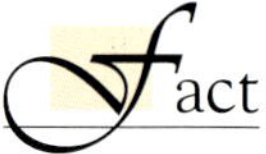

Fact

Lung cancers can arise a decade before they are even visible for the first time. Events occurring weeks or months before a diagnosis are not significant in determining outcome. This is a critical concept for patients and their physicians to understand.

When lung cancer develops, it tends to spread from the original cancer site itself to the lymph glands, and then, either at the same time or sequentially, to other areas of the body. **Figure 6** illustrates the common sites within the lung where cancer occurs. The most common sites for lung cancer spread (metastasis) are the brain, bones, liver, adrenal glands (where *adrenalin* is produced), and any other organ with a high rate of blood flow. It is this process of metastasis that leads to fatality in most patients. Therefore, when we think about lung cancer, we need to think about the symptoms caused by the primary cancer, the symptoms caused by regional metastasis within the chest, and the symptoms that may be caused by the cancer's spread to distant areas of the body.

When a physician first discovers a cancer on physical examination or on any of our diagnostic tests, it is at least 1 cm (1/2 inch) in size. Below this size, we are not quite sure, either on physical exam or on an x-ray, whether it is an abnormal finding or not.

A cancer that is 1 cm in size already contains at least 1 billion cancer cells. The time it took for that cancer to grow from 1/2 cm to 1 cm was anywhere from 3 to 5 months. If one backtracks from 1 billion, to one-half billion, to one-quarter billion, to one-eighth billion, etc., with 3- to 5-month intervals in between, it is apparent that the first malignant cells arose on the order of a decade beforehand.

FIGURE 6

Most common sites of lung cancer within the lung itself.

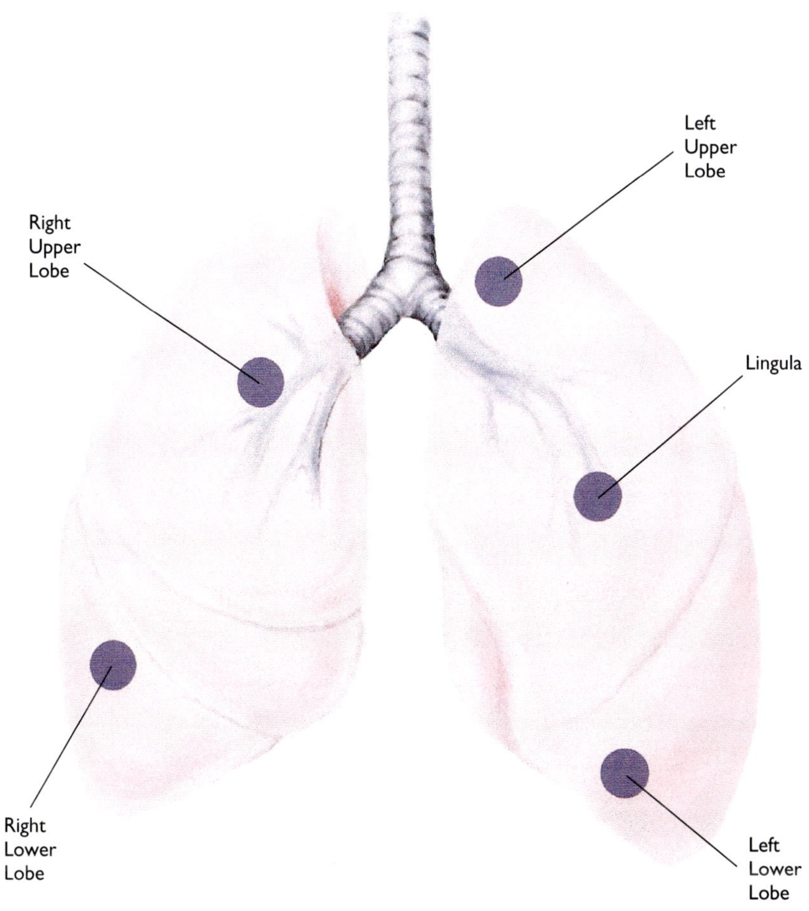

In a similar manner, when a cancer cell "learns" to spread from the primary cancer to other sites in the body, it starts as a single cell or a small clump of cells and thereafter grows just as the primary tumor grows. Occasionally, these cells will grow faster than the original cancer. Usually, however, the growth rates are relatively similar. This means that a cancer in the lung is likely to be bigger than any of the metastasized cancers.

The same problem in diagnosis occurs, however, in that a metastasis must be 1 cm to be visible on examination, or on an x-ray. Again, it took many years for that 1-cm-sized tumor to develop. There-fore, waiting a week to evaluate the characteristics and extent of the disease (a process called **staging**) is not going to result in any change in outcome. The events determining your prognosis have oc-curred years before the patient actually presented to the physician. If spread were to occur several days after the patient was initially diagnosed, it still would not be apparent for many years.

THE PHYSICAL EXAMINATION

The physical examination and diagnostic tests that follow a suspected lung cancer are all directed toward ascertaining whether the cancer is still local-ized, or whether it has become regional or distant.

Using a stethoscope, your physician will listen to the chest for any evidence of pneumonia, or col-lapse of a portion of the lung. He or she can also detect the presence of fluid in the chest cavity (pleural fluid), and, with experience, detect fluid around the heart (pericardial fluid).

Your physician will also look for signs of increased pressure on the veins in the chest, which will present as readily apparent distended neck veins. He or she will also search for spread to the lymph glands in the area just above the **clavicle** (collarbone). These glands are known as the **supraclavicular lymph nodes**. A presence of cancer in this area represents a very extensive regional spread of cancer.

During the remainder of the examination, the physician will look for signs of metastatic disease. Spread to the brain will often cause increased pressure within the skull, which results in headaches and blurred vision. The physician can detect this increased pressure when he or she looks into the back of your eye with a special light called an **ophthalmoscope**. This will allow him or her to see the veins around the optic nerve, which is a direct extension of the brain. Your physician can then assess whether there is increased pressure within the skull **(papilledema)**.

If the liver is involved with the cancer, it will often be enlarged. In this state, it can be felt by the physician, just below the rib cage on the right side.

DIAGNOSTIC TESTS

The initial history, physical examination, and chest x-ray all determine the types of diagnostic tests that will then be performed. If the physician feels that the cancer is still localized or regionalized to the chest, diagnostic tests will then be directed toward proving the patient's disease can be safely removed and cured by surgery. On the other hand, if the initial examination suggests widespread disease, diagnostic tests are then performed to rapidly verify the condition. In this case, nonsurgical therapies would be considered.

Lastly, the diagnostic tests and physical examination are used to support a process of "disaster prevention." There are many potentially serious outcomes of lung cancer, ranging from obstruction of an airway leading to pneumonia, to pressure on the spinal cord leading to paralysis. Awareness that these potentially serious outcomes are associated with lung cancer, and knowledge of their presenting features should enable a physician to diagnose them before the start of catastrophic symptoms.

Tests for Presumed Local or Regional Disease: If the patient's history, physical examination, and chest x-ray suggest local or regional disease, a series

> *"I think a second opinion is very valuable, especially if you seek out an institution that specializes in cancer and conducts cancer research. That way, you're getting the latest advances in treating your particular disease."*

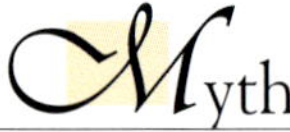

All nodules seen on chest x-ray are cancerous.

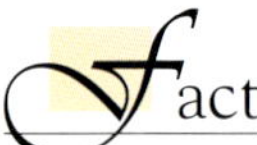

Nodules in the lungs can be due to many things. Some are **primary malignancies** arising in the lung; others are malignancies spreading from elsewhere in the body. There are, however, a number of **benign**, or noncancerous, **lesions**, including areas of old inflammation (**granulomas**), benign tumors (**hamartomas**), and other relatively benign infectious processes. The vast majority of benign lesions will be present and unchanged on chest x-ray for more than 1 year. This is *not* the case for cancer, and therefore, obtaining earlier chest x-rays is a critical part of the original evaluation.

of tests will be initiated to verify that the disease is surgically resectable and curable. The first of these tests is called a chest **CAT scan**, also known as a **CT scan** or **computed tomography**. A CT scan allows the radiologist to look inside the chest and determine whether the primary cancer is pressing against any other vital structure(s). It also identifies whether the lymph glands in the middle of the chest have been invaded. Additionally, because most CT scans include the upper abdomen, the images also suggest whether or not the cancer has affected the liver and adrenal glands.

The next most commonly performed procedure is a **bronchoscopy** (see **Figure 7**). Under local anesthesia, a flexible tube is placed down a patient's airway to search for evidence of cancer. Oftentimes, a very fine needle will be introduced into the chest to take a **biopsy (fine-needle aspiration)**.

If the CT scan and bronchoscopy still suggest that the cancer is resectable for a potential cure, two important issues will then need to be settled: 1) "Is the cancer resectable?" and 2) "Is the patient operable?"

Is the Cancer Resectable? This question refers to whether or not the cancer can be removed in its entirety. This is usually determined by assessing whether the lymph glands in the middle of the chest are involved with the cancer. Infection may cause the lymph glands to be enlarged on the CT scan, thereby making the CT scan an unreliable means of diagnosing lymph node involvement with cancer. At this point, many surgeons will perform a **mediastinoscopy**. During this procedure, a patient is placed under general anesthesia. Next, an incision is made just above the breastbone, an instrument is placed behind the breastbone, and the lymph glands are examined and biopsied. If these lymph glands prove to contain cancer, it will be almost impossible to completely resect for a cure. In this instance, nonsurgical treatments will be prescribed.

On the other hand, if these lymph glands prove to be free of cancer, a resection for cure may be quite feasible, and it is then time to proceed to the second issue.

Is the Patient Operable? The second issue entails testing to determine whether or not the patient would survive the proposed operation. The two most common causes of undue surgical risk are cardiac abnormalities and insufficient pulmonary capacity.

A patient who has recently had a *myocardial infarction* (heart attack) has an unstable heart muscle. This patient is considered to be a very high-risk candidate for further surgery before a period of several months has elapsed. Additionally, extremely high blood pressure, severe heart failure, and un-controlled *arrhythmias* (irregular heartbeats) may often preclude safe surgery until they are con-trolled. Various forms of stress tests will be per-formed if there is any question about the capacity of the heart to safely undergo surgery.

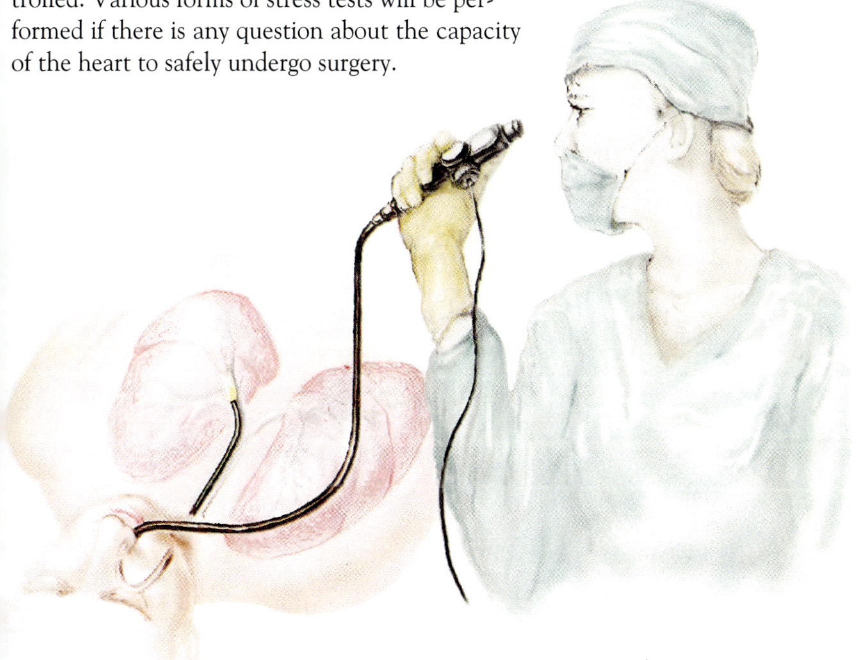

FIGURE 7

Bronchoscopy—This illustration shows the bronchoscope being fed through the nose and down the throat to the bronchus and lung.

Breathing capacity is another major determinant of patient operability. Most lung cancer patients are heavy smokers who have damaged their lungs to varying degrees. To evaluate breathing capacity, some relatively simple tests will be performed. In one, a **spirometry**, the patient breathes in and out through a mouthpiece into an instrument. A spirometry lets the physician know how much lung capacity remains, and whether or not the proposed removal of lung tissue, along with the tumor, would leave a safe amount of normal lung tissue to allow for normal breathing.

When simple breathing tests reveal marginal pulmonary function, several more sophisticated breathing tests can be performed for further evaluation. In this instance, it is advisable to be seen at a center with physicians who are skilled at complex, high-risk surgical procedures.

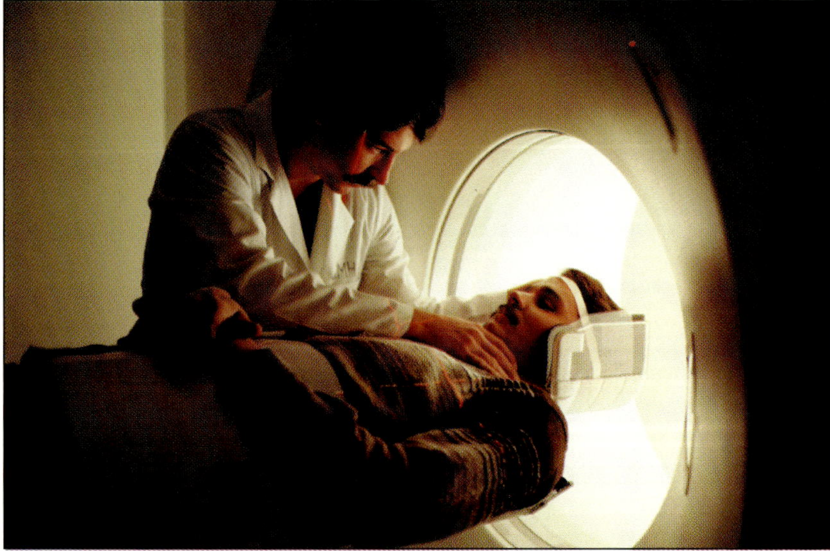

FIGURE 8

©*PhotoDisc*

Magnetic resonance imaging (MRI) of a patient's brain: The patient lies comfortably on what may be a cushioned surface, and his head is fitted into a soft cushion. A machine will produce a strong magnetic field along with low-energy radio waves, which will then detail images of the body, regardless of intervening bone.

Tests for Presumed Distant (Widespread) Disease: If the initial studies reveal that the patient may have widespread disease, it makes no sense to perform complex tests to determine whether a patient can be safely resected. Instead, the most rapid and definitive procedure should be performed to confirm distant disease. As part of the initial work-up, a set of blood tests will be performed. One of them, the **alkaline phosphatase**, is often a harbinger of spread to the liver or bone. The liver is usually well visualized on the CT scan of the chest. If the liver is normal on CT scan, but the alkaline phosphatase level is elevated, a bone scan should be obtained, even if there are no symptoms of spread to the bone.

Bone pain, too, should be investigated with a **bone scan**. A bone scan involves the injection of a mildly radioactive phosphorus into newly forming bone. Wherever a cancer destroys a bone, the body tries to repair the bone directly next to it and it is this repair process that shows up on the bone scan. A symptom of back pain could also indicate the presence of a condition known as **bony metastasis**. Here, the possible compression of the spinal cord by a tumor is not well diagnosed by the bone scan or routine x-rays. An MRI of the spine is the definitive way to be sure that bony metastasis is not present.

In the presence of headaches, double vision, and/or confusion, the preferred test is a **magnetic resonance imaging (MRI)** of the brain **(Figure 8)**. Often, a CT scan of the head with contrast is substituted; but it is not quite as effective.

Obviously, symptoms related to any other organ are pursued with tests specific for that organ, whether they be CT scans or other **dye-contrast studies**. Unfortunately, there are no specific blood tests for lung cancer. Occasionally, one of the "**tumor markers**," such as CEA (carcinoembryonic antigen), will be elevated in lung cancer, but because this is neither diagnostic nor particularly useful, it is not routinely ordered.

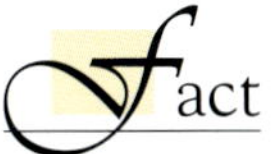

*M*yth

If my chest x-ray is read as negative, I don't have lung cancer.

*F*act

Chest x-rays often miss lung cancers, which can hide as small shadows behind the ribs or behind the vascular structures in the middle of the chest.

Lung Cancer Staging—Its Definition and Significance

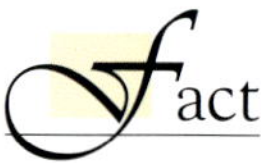

Myth

My surgeon said he removed all of my cancer.

Fact

Other than the very earliest and smallest lung cancers, it is quite unusual for the surgeon to "remove all of the cancer." It is vital that the full extent of the disease and all aspects of the staging process be ascertained before embarking on a course of therapy.

In the Diagnosis chapter, we discussed the various ways to determine whether or not a patient has local, regional (locally advanced), or distant (widespread) disease. The process of evaluating all the characteristics of a cancer is called **staging**. The physician must assign these stages in an orderly, accurate fashion in order to garner a correct prognosis and therapy selection.

Staging is classified by **T stage**, which describes a tumor's characteristics; **N stage**, which determines the extent of lymph node involvement; and **M stage**, which denotes the presence or absence of metastasis. Grouping the T, N, and M status of a patient's lung cancer enables the physician to identify the stage of a cancer by number (Stage 1, Stage 2, Stage 3, Stage 4). Each number designates a T, N, and M grouping.

T STAGE

The extent of the local tumor is dependent on two basic factors, first the size of the tumor, and second, whether or not the tumor involves adjacent vital structures. **Figure 9** depicts T-stage cancers.

- A Tx cancer is a tumor that is proven to exist because of the presence of malignant cells in the bronchopulmonary secretions. This type of tumor, however, cannot be visualized on any test. A Tx tumor is also known as a tumor that cannot be assessed.

- A T1 cancer is a cancer that is less than 3 cm (1^1/$_2$ in) in size and completely surrounded by lung tissue.

• A T2 cancer is any cancer larger than 3 cm still surrounded by lung tissue, and not invading the chest wall or any of the structures in the middle of the chest.

• A T3 cancer is a cancer of any size that invades the chest wall or the structures of the chest's center. A T3 cancer is still completely and safely

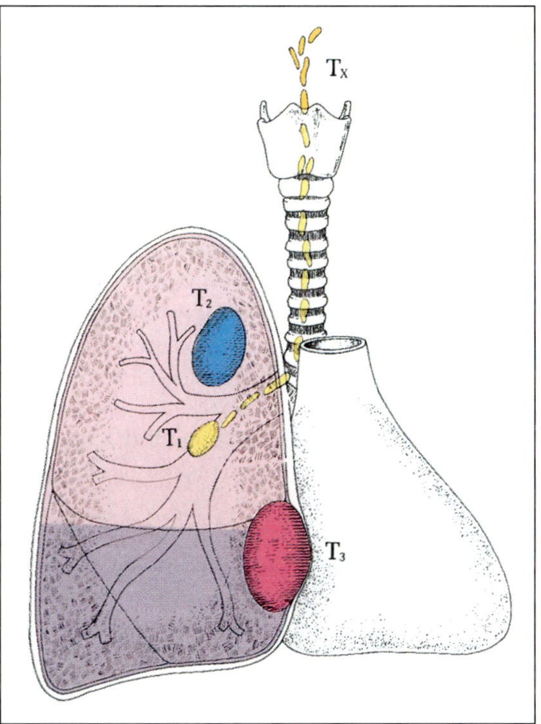

FIGURE 9

*An artist's depiction of 4 different T-stage cancers. Tx refers to the proven presence of a tumor by certain secretions, yet one that cannot be visualized during any test; it also refers to any tumor that cannot be assessed. T1 is defined as a tumor measuring 3 cm or less, surrounded by lung or pleura, and without evidence of invasion to a bronchus. T2 illustrates a tumor measuring more than 3 cm, or a tumor of any size that either invades the pleura or has **atelectasis** or **obstructive pneumonitis**. A T4 tumor may be of any size with invasion into the mediastinum; or a tumor that involves the heart, great vessels, trachea, esophagus, vertebral body or carina, or a presence of malignant pleural effusion.*

resectable, because the operation can be performed around the area of the cancer.

• A T4 cancer is a tumor of any size that invades vital structures, such as the soft tissues of the mediastinum and the vertebral body. It cannot be removed safely, and hence, is definitively unresectable. The windpipe flows down the chest from the neck, and divides into two tubes (called bronchi) (see **Figure 1** on page 14) that direct the flow of air to each lung. The area where these two bronchi diverge from each other is called the carina. If a cancer is too close to the **carina**, the surgeon cannot safely sew the remaining airways together. As a result, these particular T4 cancers—even when they are relatively small—may also be unresectable. Any individual with a T4 cancer that is being considered for resection should be seen at a major cancer center that performs a large number of these procedures.

N STAGE

The lymph nodes—or outposts of the immune system—are spread throughout the body. Normally, fragments of bacteria, viruses, eroded normal cells, and other foreign bodies are carried to the nearest lymph node, then analyzed by the body's immune system. When they are foreign, we develop an immune reaction against them; when they are normal breakdown products, they are ignored. Unfortunately, a cancer cell is perceived by the body's immune system as a normal cell, and therefore, it is ignored. Consequently, the extent of lymph node involvement provides a sense of how long the tumor has had the capacity to metastasize.

Within the chest, the lymph nodes are broken down into three major areas; the **hilar lymph nodes**, the **mediastinal lymph nodes**, and the supraclavicular lymph nodes. (See **Figure 5** on page 25.)

As the airway, or bronchus, branches off the windpipe into each side of the chest, the lung is fitted around the end of it, somewhat like a balloon. The area at the neck of the balloon is called the **hilum** of the lung, and the lymph nodes in this area are called the hilar lymph nodes. The mediastinal lymph nodes are defined as the lymph nodes that exist in the middle of the chest in and among the windpipe and esophagus. These nodes can exist on the same side that the cancer arose *(ipsilateral)*, or on the other side *(contralateral)*. The third lymph node station, called the supraclavicular area, exists just above the collarbones. A presence of cancer in either the hilar lymph nodes, the mediastinal lymph nodes, or the supraclavicular area is considered indicative of a regional spread of lung cancer. Any lymph nodes involved beyond this area (for example further up in the neck or under the arms) are considered indicative of distant (widespread) disease.

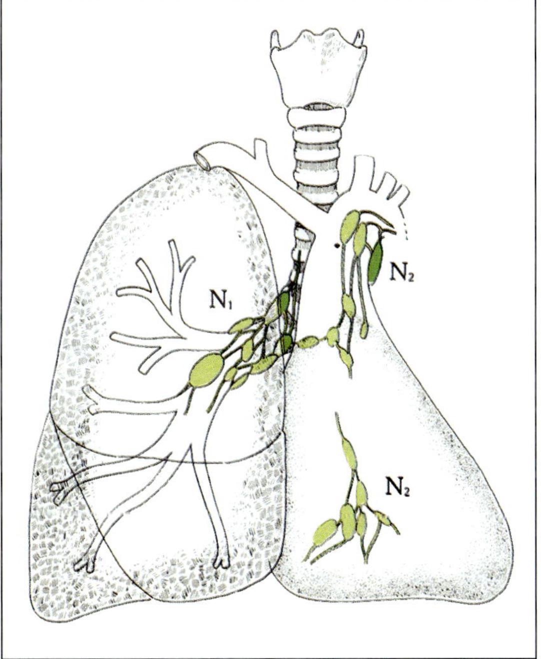

FIGURE 10

*An artist's depiction of N1 and N2 nodal involvement. N1 illustrates a metastasis of the **intrapulmonary** lymph nodes; N2 shows metastasis to the ipsilateral lymph nodes and the subcarinal lymph nodes.*

Lymph node involvement in lung cancer is identified by N stage. **Figure 10** illustrates both an N1 and N2 nodal involvement.

The definitions for each N stage are as follows:
- N0 refers to the absence of any lymph node involvement.
- N1 refers to the presence of cancer in the hilar lymph nodes. Some of these hilar lymph nodes can actually exist within the main tissue of the lung itself.
- N2 refers to an involvement of the mediastinal lymph nodes on the cancer side.
- N3 cancers involve the lymph nodes on the other side of the chest, or in the supraclavicular area.

The more extensive the lymph node involvement, the higher the likelihood that the cancer has spread beyond the chest into other organs throughout the body.

M STAGE

The M stage is used to identify the presence of metastasis; its staging system is somewhat simpler than the T and N groups.
- M0 implies the absence of any evidence of cancer spread to other organs.
- M1 implies cancer spread to any organ.

In clinical research, it is often important to distinguish between cancer spread to a single site outside of the chest and spread to multiple, distant sites. Spread to multiple sites is never associated with a cure. There are unusual, but well-reported, instances of spread to single sites, particularly the brain. In this case, an aggressive local approach to removing the isolated brain metastasis and treating the isolated lung cancer will result in cure for the patient. However, these are very unusual circumstances and will be addressed in more detail later.

STAGES I THROUGH 4

Lung cancer is also broken down into four different stages, several of which have subcategories. Although imperfect, this staging system provides a good understanding of the prognosis of lung cancer.

FIGURE 11

The most common sites for lung cancer metastases are the brain, bones, liver, adrenal glands, and any other organ with a high rate of blood flow.

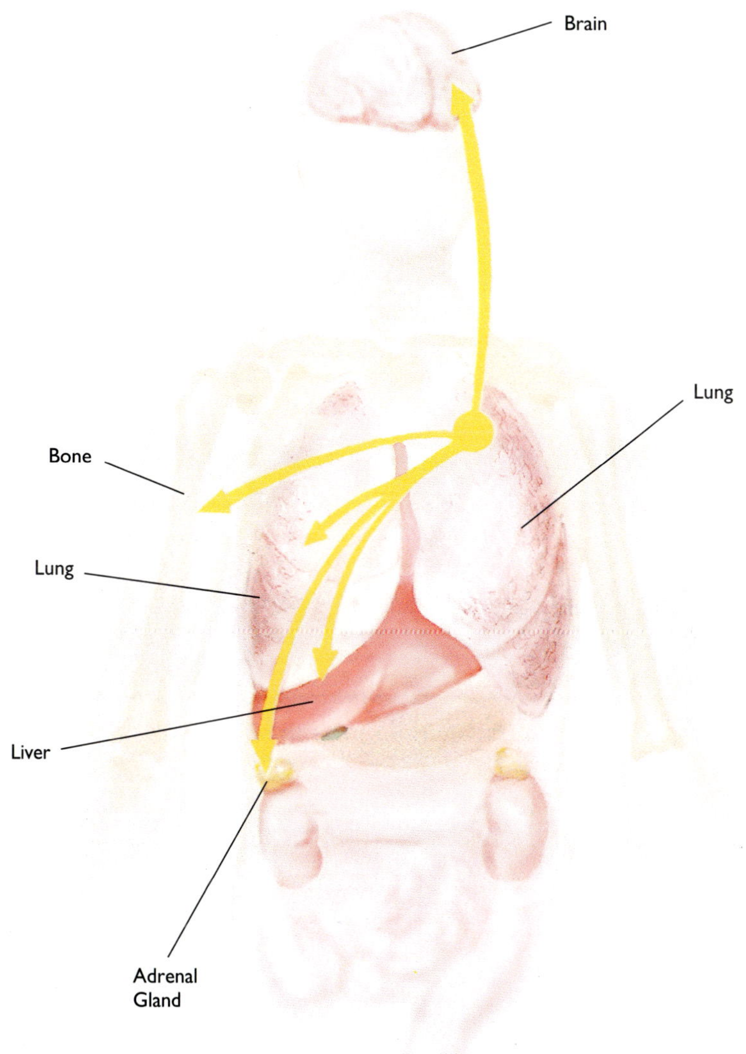

This system also provides physicians with the information they will need to choose the most rational therapy for their patients.

Stage 1 Disease: Stage 1 disease is characterized by an absence of cancer spread to any lymph node whatsoever. Stage 1A disease implies a very small cancer without lymph node involvement. Stage 1B disease is a larger cancer without lymph node involvement.

Stage 2 Disease: Stage 2A and 2B disease fundamentally refers to the presence of cancer in the hilar lymph nodes, or N1 area, in addition to the primary site in the lung. The presence of a tumor involving the chest wall without hilar lymph node involvement (T3, N0) is also recognized as Stage 2B disease. These tumors can be safely removed and surgically cured by cutting around the malignant involvement in the chest wall, hence reverting the cancer back to a Stage 2B instead of Stage 3.

Stage 3 Disease: Stage 3 disease is broken down into two major categories: Stage 3A and Stage 3B disease. Stage 3A disease involves the mediastinal lymph glands on the same side as the cancer. This cancer may either be resectable initially or following preoperative treatment. In patients with Stage 3B disease, there is lymph node involvement on the other side of the chest, or in the supraclavicular area (N3). These patients should never be considered for surgical resection.

Stage 4 Disease: Stage 4 disease implies that the cancer has spread outside of the chest. **Figure 11** illustrates the most common sites for lung cancer metastases. The staging system is somewhat inadequate regarding the interface between Stage 3B and Stage 4 disease. In patients with tumor cells involving the lining around the lung, along with fluid production in that space (a ***malignant pleural effusion***), the disease is not curable by any combination of surgery and ***radiation therapy (local therapies)***. Their disease behaves more like Stage 4 disease, and yet the staging system considers them Stage 3B. Most clinicians, however, do consider these patients Stage 4.

Non-Small-Cell Lung Cancer

As discussed earlier, the small-cell lung cancers derived from the hormonal cells of the lung have traditionally behaved differently than all other forms of cancer known as non-small-cell lung cancer. Although these differences are less apparent today, we will discuss the staging procedures and treatment options for small-cell lung cancer in the following chapter. Here, we will focus on the staging system and treatment of non-small-cell lung cancer.

TREATING STAGE I NON-SMALL-CELL LUNG CANCER

The primary treatment for Stage 1 disease is surgery. As outlined earlier, however, a patient's cancer must first be defined as "resectable" (that is, readily removable for a potential cure) and "operable" (such that the patient will survive the operation). If these two conditions are met, a Stage 1A cancer can be treated with surgery alone and cured somewhere between 65% and 80% of the time. However, due to the cancer's ability to microscopically spread quite early in the cancer's course, even these small cancers have a recognizable *recurrence* rate.

With surgical therapy alone, Stage 1B disease has a cure rate of approximately 50%. Several studies are now exploring whether chemotherapy administered before or after surgery is beneficial in reducing the number of recurrences. This issue, however, has not yet been resolved.

It cannot be stressed enough that all of the chest's lymph nodes must be examined prior to surgery. Thereafter, the lymph nodes must either be removed or sampled before surgery (at mediastinos-

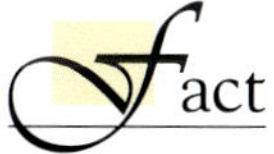

Myth

Chemotherapy is not worthwhile for the patient with advanced lung cancer.

Fact

There have been significant improvements in chemotherapy in recent years. Combination regimens can increase survival duration in some patients with advanced disease. Plus the availability of improved agents and drugs to reduce or avoid side effects like nausea and vomiting have made chemotherapy more tolerable.

copy) or during surgery. If this procedure is not performed, both the stage and curative potential of the surgical procedure will be unknown. Some surgeons who are less experienced in the management of lung cancer assume they can tell whether or not a lymph node is involved with cancer by feeling the lymph node with their gloved finger during the operation. This misconception often causes missed diagnoses of microscopic disease.

Four basic operations are performed for all Stage 1 non-small-cell lung cancers:

- a **pneumonectomy**, where the entire lung is removed,
- a **lobectomy**, where one portion (a lobe) is removed,
- a **limited resection**, where one subportion (a segment or wedge) is removed, and
- a **sleeve resection**, where a section of intervening lung is removed.

Removal of the entire lung (pneumonectomy) was once the most common operation for lung cancer; but this is not usually the case today.

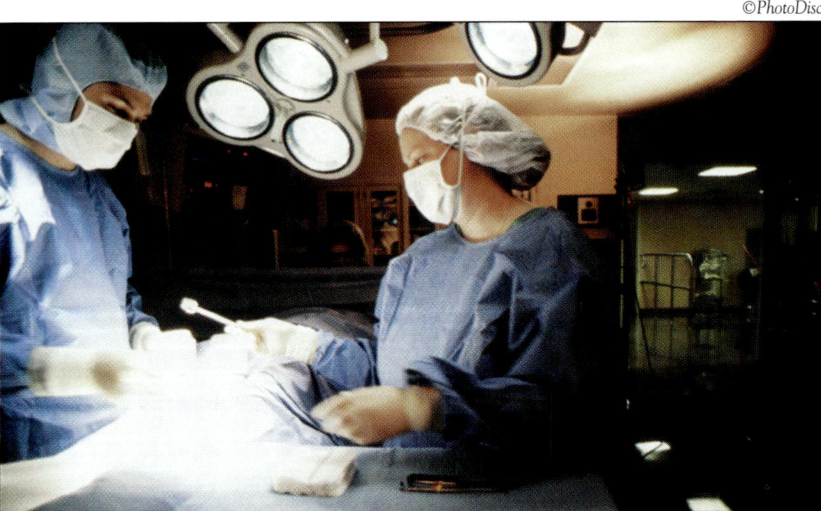

The primary treatment for Stage 1 disease is surgery. However, a patient's cancer must first be defined as "resectable" and "operable."

Limited resections are helpful for removing a minimal amount of lung tissue in patients with very marginal or borderline breathing function. They should not, however, substitute for the removal of a full lobe (lobectomy) when that operation can be safely performed. When a lung cancer arises quite close to the carina, an operation called a sleeve resection can often be performed. During this difficult operation, a section of intervening lung is removed and the more distant portion of the lung is then reattached to the main airway. All sleeve resections are considered difficult and should therefore be performed in centers with experience.

TREATING STAGE 2 NON-SMALL-CELL LUNG CANCER

Stage 2 disease is characterized by a lung cancer that has affected the hilar lymph nodes. Like Stage 1 cancers, Stage 2 cancers are also potentially curable by surgery—although the cure rates now fall to approximately 30% to 40%. This holds true for Stage 2A and Stage 2B diseases, as well. Numerous studies have attempted to explore whether radiation, chemotherapy, or both, can be added to surgical resection in Stage 2 disease. Some evidence suggests that adding chemotherapy provides a small benefit; approximately 4% more patients are alive at 5 years with this addition. Recent evidence suggests, however, that giving radiation therapy to patients with resected N1 disease is *not* helpful, and may in fact even be harmful. This issue is not yet clear. If postoperative radiation therapy for Stage 2 disease is proposed, you should seek a second opinion.

Controversy exists over whether or not to radiate a T3 N0 lung cancer that has involved the chest wall. Most treatment teams will use radiation therapy if this cancer has invaded the muscle or ribs. However, to date, no definitive studies have confirmed the efficacy of this procedure.

TREATING STAGE 3 NON-SMALL-CELL LUNG CANCER

The biggest whir of controversy undoubtedly revolves around the treatment of Stage 3A disease. For a long period of time, patients with any evidence of mediastinal lymph node involvement were considered unresectable and referred for radiation therapy. Today, it has become clear that some patients with very limited N2 disease can be cured with surgery alone; however, the proportion of these patients is quite small. Preoperative or postoperative chemotherapy and radiation seem to improve the outcome in these patients.

In recent years, most studies have focused on preoperative, or so-called **neoadjuvant**, therapy. Even though the benefit of preoperative therapy is not yet proven, this procedure is widely used. This important question regarding the value of preoperative therapy is now being considered in clinical trials; at a minimum, we recommend that any person being considered for preoperative therapy obtain a second opinion.

In the past, patients with Stage 3B disease were treated with radiation therapy alone. Several studies now suggest that chemotherapy before, or along with radiation therapy, improves the outcome for patients with Stage 3B disease. However, various clinical studies are still evaluating the exact sequence, dosing schedule, and choice of chemotherapy. Some evidence suggests that radiation therapy administered more than once a day may also improve results. Radiation therapy can, in fact, be given in more than one session (**fraction**) per day—a technique known as **hyperfractionation**. Thereafter, these fractions are carried out over the same total length of treatment. Shortening the overall length of the treatment is called accelerated radiation. The combination of hyperfractionation and accelerated radiation is known as hyperfractionated accelerated radiation. This may offer some enhancements to survival that are equivalent to chemotherapy plus radiation. Hyperfractionation, accelerated radiation, and hyperfractionated accelerated radiation with and without chemotherapy are currently under study.

TREATING STAGE 4 NON-SMALL-CELL LUNG CANCER

Active treatment for Stage 4 disease involves chemotherapy. Prior to initiating chemotherapy, however, two criteria need to be met. First, the patient needs to decide whether an attempt at treatment to prolong life (but not cure his or her disease) is preferable to an approach that will only treat symptoms (*palliative care*).

The vast majority of patients do choose chemotherapy, but all patients should explore this decision with their physicians. I like to phrase the implied contract with a patient in this way: "We will aggressively treat to prolong your life, but not to prolong your suffering." This becomes a very individualized decision for each patient and his or her family and physician.

The second requirement is that the patient be medically fit to tolerate chemotherapy. Clinicians determine this using a *performance status scale*—a critically important test that can determine whether patients will tolerate chemotherapy (**Table 3**).

TABLE 3

Performance Status	Description
0	No symptoms at all, capable of normal activities
1	Some symptoms, but able to carry on most activities
2	Symptomatic, requiring a nap or return to bed for up to half the day
3	Symptomatic and fatigued enough to spend more than half the day in bed
4	Bedridden

Performance status 0 and 1 patients will tolerate chemotherapy quite normally and will generally not have serious side effects. Patients with performance status 3 and 4 will rarely, if ever, respond to chemotherapy; most often, it only worsens their overall condition. For these patients, palliative care to keep them comfortable might be preferred. More problematic, however, is a performance status of 2. These patients return to bed for an hour or two nap every afternoon because they are fatigued from their cancer. They may feel reasonably well when they are up and about, but they do not tolerate chemotherapy as well as patients with a performance status of 0 or 1. The proscriptions against treatment in this group are not so strong, however, that an individualized decision cannot be made. In general, if the patient takes a brief nap but feels strongly that he or she would like to try chemotherapy, the therapy should be attempted. On the other hand, the patient who sleeps 49% of the day and is hardly awake the rest of the day might not benefit from chemotherapy. Nonetheless, the boundary between these two extremes needs to be fully absorbed and comprehended by each patient and his or her family and physician.

CHEMOTHERAPY FOR NON-SMALL-CELL LUNG CANCER

It is interesting to note that most people believe chemotherapy involves radiation. In fact, chemotherapy, simply put, is the treatment of disease by chemical agents. Most often, the chemotherapeutic agent, or drug, is injected into the bloodstream by either a needle or catheter.

Chemotherapy for non-small-cell lung cancer has had a bad name for many years. Initially, this was because it made virtually no impact on the cancer. In the 1980s, however, newer compounds arrived and physicians began to witness a prolongation of life from chemotherapy. Yet, because of the side effects of extreme nausea and vomiting, it was hard to tell whether it was worthwhile to continue with therapy. Since the early 1990s, though, an influx of improved chemotherapy agents and **anti-emetics** (drugs that prevent or lessen the associated side effects of nausea and vomiting) have made chemotherapy for non-small-cell lung cancers very tolerable. An assessment of whether chemotherapy will be active against the cancer can now be made without the issue of overwhelming side effects.

New Drugs: In the mid 1990s, a whole series of new drugs became available: **paclitaxel (Taxol)**, **gemcitabine (Gemzar)**, and **vinorelbine (Navelbine)**. These agents yielded a much-improved series of side effects compared to older compounds, including less nausea and vomiting.

Throughout the mid 1990s, combination regimens using older and newer compounds have resulted in what appears to be a significant improvement in the number of patients responding to chemotherapy. These combinations have also significantly improved patients' length of survival. For information about these chemotherapy agents, you should speak to your medical oncologist.

The efficacy of this **combination chemotherapy**, or **polychemotherapy**, is an area that is very important for patients and their family members to understand. One way to talk about the results of therapy is to discuss the average, or the median, survival. If a particular therapy produces a response rate and long-term survival in more than 50% of patients, this way of describing outcome can be helpful. When less than one half of the patients are so affected, the use of median survival may be misleading.

We clinicians, however, like to rely more on the proportion of patients who are alive at 1 or 2 years following the initiation of chemotherapy. If no chemotherapy is given to a patient with metastatic non-small-cell lung cancer, or none of the therapies succeeds, the average survival will be about 6 months, and only 10% of these patients will be alive

> *"Family members are always wondering, 'Have I done enough?' It was important to me to have my doctor talk to my family and include them in the learning process."*

at 1 year. With some of the earlier chemotherapies, the proportion of patients who responded to the chemotherapy was only 25% to 30%—the average survival didn't surpass 8 or 9 months. However, given today's improved chemotherapy drugs, the proportion of patients alive at 1 year rose to 25%, and a recognizable, although small, proportion of patients (approximately 5%) lived 2 years.

Studies have shown that when the newer drugs were used in combination with one of the older compounds, nearly 50% of patients responded to therapy. With these combination regimens, the average survival was over 1 year. Hence, 50% of patients lived for 1 year, and nearly 20% lived for 2 years (with small numbers living for an even longer period of time). Although this combination chemo-therapy is hardly the definitive answer for treatment of metastatic non-small-cell lung cancer, it is, nonetheless, a significant improvement from where we were just a few years ago. Whether or not the degree of benefit outweighs the side effects of com-bination therapy is a decision that should be made by the individual patient and his or her family and physician. The discussion should occur, however, with a physician who is experienced in the use of chemotherapy—a medical oncologist.

Small-Cell Lung Cancer

From the very earliest studies of lung cancer, it was clear that small-cell lung cancer tended to spread earlier and grow faster than all non-small-cell lung cancers. Consequently, very early in its history, small-cell lung cancer was designated as a disease that was always approached in a nonsurgical manner. Because chemotherapy solely attacks growing, dividing cells, the rapidly dividing small-cell lung cancers were, of course, more responsive to chemotherapy. Patients with disease limited to the chest were felt to be curable upwards of 25% of the time with chemotherapy and radiation. To date, however, those numbers have somewhat improved, yet the proportion cured still has not risen very far above 35%. It has been reported that a tiny fraction of patients with extensive disease have been cured.

Let's look at the facts about small-cell lung cancer.

TWO PRESENTATIONS OF SMALL-CELL LUNG CANCER: LIMITED AND EXTENSIVE

Although we can use the same staging system for both small-cell lung and non-small-cell lung cancers, a tradition has arisen whereby small-cell lung cancers are described as either **"limited"** or **"extensive."** This is a historical aberration; nonetheless, it persists in clinical treatment.

Limited Small-Cell Lung Cancer: Limited small-cell lung cancer refers to a cancer that is confined to the chest. Colloquially, it is defined as a disease that can be encompassed within a single radiation treatment area or port. The fact that such a port would be impractical for treatment is not usually taken into account in this staging system, and there is a great deal of disagreement about the specifics of

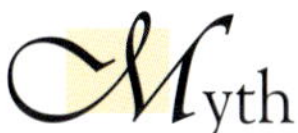

Even though small-cell lung cancer is a faster growing cancer, it is the only truly curable form of lung cancer.

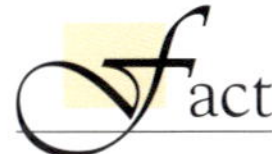

Stage for stage, small-cell lung cancer behaves about the same as non-small-cell lung cancer. In part, this is due to significant improvements in chemotherapy for non-small-cell lung cancers versus the absence of progress in the treatment of small-cell lung cancer.

the term, "limited." People argue about whether lymph node spread to the area above the clavicle (supraclavicular area) on the unaffected side of the chest is limited or extensive disease.

Extensive Small-Cell Lung Cancer: Extensive small-cell lung cancer refers to any degree of cancer spread beyond the chest. The same staging procedures used to search for the presence or absence of non-small-cell lung cancer are used for small-cell lung cancer. The same philosophy of staging holds true, as well: If the history and physical examination suggest no evidence of distant disease, then tests are performed to provide confirmation that the disease is confined to the chest and that the patient's lungs can tolerate aggressive radiation and chemotherapy. On the other hand, the presence of symptoms suggestive of widespread disease calls for the most rapid test to search for the site of metastasis.

TREATING SMALL-CELL LUNG CANCER

Over the past 2 or 3 decades, several regimens were used for the treatment of small-cell lung cancer. In the late 1980s, a new combination regimen forged to the forefront and has since become a standard treatment for small-cell lung cancer.

Several studies are currently evaluating the effects of adding one or more of the newer agents to the basic regimen used today. However, it is not yet clear whether any of these combination chemotherapies will prove to be superior. Countless studies have attempted to pinpoint the optimal dosage; they have increased dosages, added to dosages, provided drugs as maintenance therapies or **prophylactic therapies**, or delivered higher dosages following a standard-dose therapy (**late intensification**). However, not one of these techniques has proven to be successful in improving the basic response and survival rates that were achieved with the basic regimen.

Treating Limited Small-Cell Lung Cancer: Limited small-cell lung cancer is treated with chemotherapy and radiation. Most investigators believe

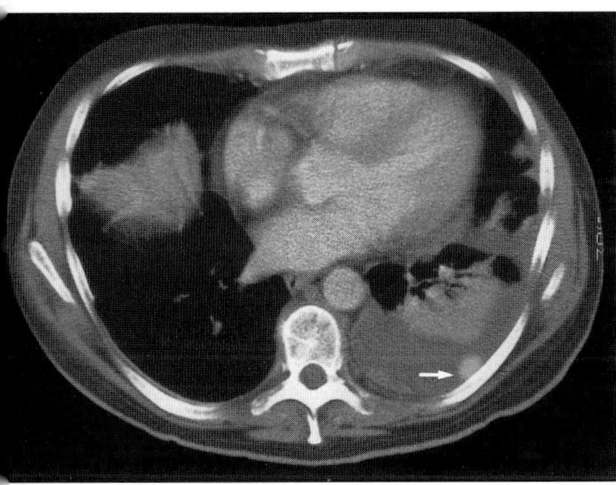

FIGURE 12

Malignant Pleural Effusion—A single CT slice shows a malignant, left-sided pleural effusion in this patient with adenocarcinoma of the lungs. Note the tumor nodule (arrow).

that radiation therapy and chemotherapy should be administered concurrently—with the radiation being initiated as early in the course of chemotherapy as possible. Delaying radiation therapy until the end of several months of chemotherapy appears to be somewhat less effective. Current studies are trying to determine whether radiation therapy should be administered once or twice a day. To date, however, there have been no significant differences in outcome—although some increase in side effects was noted with radiation therapy administered twice a day.

Occasionally, physicians will find a small nodule on the patient's chest x-ray and proceed to the evaluation. If the lesion is quite small and there is no evidence of lymph node involvement on the CT scan, surgery would be the next option. In turn, surgery may reveal that the cancer is a very early small-cell lung cancer. Sometimes, a biopsy before surgery will uncover a small-cell anaplastic cancer. Again, as long as the lesion is quite small and there is no evidence of lymph node involvement on the CT scan, a surgical approach appears to be warranted.

It is our belief that if a diagnosis of small-cell lung cancer is determined prior to surgery, the physician should then carefully assess the mediastinum—even proceeding to a **mediastinoscopy** (surgical evaluation of the mediastinum). This surgical approach would then be followed by 4 to 6 cycles of standard chemotherapy. This subgroup of patients proves to have a very high cure rate. Approximately 50% to 75% of patients will be cured following surgery and chemotherapy for these very localized small-cell lung cancers.

Treating Extensive Small-Cell Lung Cancer: In patients with extensive disease, chemotherapy is presently the sole form of treatment. With chemotherapy, approximately 5% of patients with extensive disease may be cured. Any response to chemotherapy, short of a **complete response** (denoting no evidence of disease), however, does not have a strong impact on survival. One category of extensive small-cell lung cancer appears to behave similarly to limited disease. This category includes patients with evidence of cancer spread to the **pleura** (lining around the inside of the chest), called a malignant pleural effusion (**Figure 12**). When this effusion is confined to one side of the chest, patients seem to fare as well as patients with limited disease.

NUANCES OF SMALL-CELL LUNG CANCER

Small-cell lung cancers contain a few nuances, the first of which is the incidence of unsuspected spread to the brain. This type of metastasis is substantially higher for small-cell lung cancer patients than non-small-cell lung cancer patients. Consequently, an MRI of the brain (or a contrasted CT scan) is a requirement of the staging process for small-cell-lung cancer, regardless of whether the patient has symptoms suggestive of metastasis to the brain.

For many years, it was also believed that the incidence of spread to the bone marrow (as opposed to the bone itself) was significantly higher for small-cell lung cancer patients. Consequently, a **bone marrow aspiration** and biopsy were often included as routine tests in the staging work up for small-cell lung cancer. It now appears, however, that the incidence of such spread to the bone marrow in the absence of spread elsewhere is so low that this procedure is no longer warranted.

Brain Metastases: There is a high incidence of brain metastases in patients whose small-cell lung cancer has gone into remission elsewhere in the body. In these specific patients, the brain's blood vessels contain special cells that create a *"blood-brain barrier."* This barrier prevents chemotherapy from entering the brain as efficiently as it does elsewhere in the body.

Over the years, numerous studies have tried to assess the benefits of utilizing **prophylactic cranial irradiation** to the brain following chemotherapy and radiation. The data, however, show it has no benefit unless given to patients who are in a complete response. In these patients, the evidence to date suggests that prophylactic irradiation garners a very small improvement in overall survival. Moreover, recurrences within the brain as a first site of progression have been markedly reduced. The treatment of established brain metastasis is not a perfect science, and patients are often left with significant neurological defects. Consequently, in most instances, physicians will only recommend prophylactic cranial irradiation to patients with limited small-cell lung cancers who appear to be in complete remission following chemotherapy and radiation.

A patient with extensive disease with a complete disappearance of his or her cancer on x-ray studies is also a candidate for prophylactic cranial irradiation. The only caveat is that cranial irradiation causes both short- and long-term **cognitive dysfunction** (loss of memory and analytic ability). For most individuals, this is minor and barely noticeable, but for those whose work involves a fair

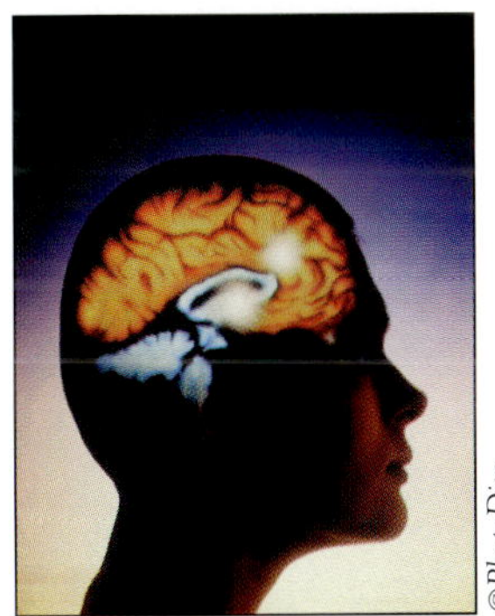

The incidence of unsuspected spread to the brain is substantially higher for small-cell lung cancer patients.

degree of analytic reasoning, this may prove to be unacceptable. In addition, individuals with early signs of **dementia** or a strong family history of dementia may more poorly tolerate brain irradiation.

Carcinoid and Atypical Carcinoid Tumors: As noted earlier, small-cell lung cancers are derived from the hormonal cells in the lung. Technically, they are referred to as small-cell, anaplastic lung cancers, the term, anaplastic, meaning "wildly growing."

There are distinct variations of these types of hormonally derived tumors. In their most differentiated state, these cells are called **carcinoid tumors**. Oftentimes, these carcinoid tumors will arise in the small intestine, but they can also originate in the lung. If they are true carcinoid tumors, they will behave quite benignly and should be surgically resected. If by chance they later recur and spread, they are treated like small-cell lung cancer. Regrettably, therapy results are less positive in carcinoid tumors that metastasize.

Under the microscope, a middle group of cancers appear to be, and look like, carcinoid tumors. These are usually labeled "atypical carcinoids." To date, it is not quite clear how to treat a very localized, atypical carcinoid tumor. When it appears as a single nodule, physicians will often surgically treat it almost as if it were a more benign form. On the other hand,

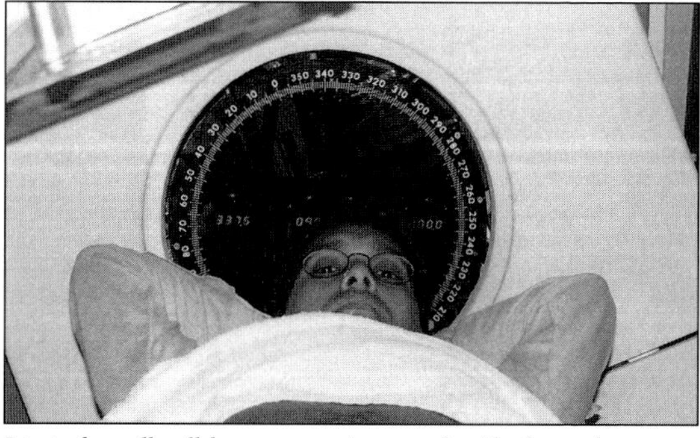

Limited small-cell lung cancer is treated with chemotherapy and radiation.

if the physician finds that the atypical carcinoid has spread to any of the lymph glands (or, of course, anywhere else in the body), he or she will treat it like its very similar cousin, small-cell lung cancer.

VACCINE AND GENE THERAPIES FOR SMALL-CELL LUNG CANCER

Small-cell lung cancers were the first lung cancers to be grown in tissue culture, as well as the first lung cancer to be biologically understood. Vaccines have been developed for treatment following the attainment of remission. Several attempts have also been made to develop antibodies or medications (vaccines) that interfere with the various growth factors that small-cell lung cancers need to grow. In addition, several gene therapy protocols that attempt to *trick* the body's immune system into believing the small-cell-lung cancer is foreign have been developed. If you are interested in this form of therapy, you may wish to consider referral to a research institution; however, the results of vaccine and gene therapies are not yet superior to standard therapy. They are, nonetheless, an exciting approach for the future.

The Follow-Up Treatment of Lung Cancer

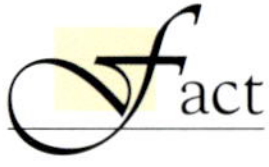

Myth

Any ache or pain that develops following the treatment of lung cancer should be considered a possible sign of recurrence.

Fact

Lung cancer can certainly recur in almost any site of the body. Most lung cancer patients are older and will consequently have the aches and pains that are common to being "over 39." Usually, physicians consider the presence of new symptoms, a persistent increase in symptoms, or unexplained weight loss as indicators that a recurrent cancer may be present.

During the lung cancer patient's follow-up period, three major factors will be analyzed:

- Evaluating the effect of the original treatment
- Monitoring for recurrence of the original cancer
- Keeping an eye out for the development of *second primary cancers*

THE FOLLOW-UP EXAMINATION

When a lung cancer patient has completed active treatment, several measures are evaluated during the follow-up. During therapy, your physician will have looked for the most easily measurable disease. He or she may have looked for a lymph gland that can be felt and measured or a suspicious finding on chest x-ray. Your physician may have also required a CT scan of the chest to elucidate the size of an individual lesion. The size of this lesion will then be analyzed during subsequent studies. Therefore, follow-up for initial response is carried out by repeating the same tests that best measured the illness when treatment first started. Obviously, if new symptoms develop at another site, specific tests to diagnose any potential problems will be ordered.

Next, the original cancer is measured in the most convenient way, and then followed most often with either a chest x-ray or a CT scan of the chest. Certain blood tests have also been reported to be helpful in this regard.

Most physicians will study a patient on a monthly basis. At the end of all therapy, he or she will then perform what is called a "restaging evaluation."

Because physicians are familiar with lung cancer sites of metastasis, an MRI of the brain, a bone scan, and CT scan of the chest and upper abdomen will often be used as a baseline for further follow-up. At this time, a routine chest x-ray, as well as a complete history and physical examination, will also be taken.

After the restaging evaluation, patients are then followed quarterly. For the first year, a patient will be called in every 3 months for a chest x-ray, history, and physical examination. After the first year, these tests will then be administered semi-annually, and thereafter, annually unless there is evidence of recurrence. During a routine follow-up of a patient in remission, a physician will only obtain a chest x-ray and routine blood tests—unless the patient develops unexplained weight loss, a new area of pain, or signs and symptoms of spread to the bone or brain. In these instances, a full array of studies specific to those sites of potential abnormality will be performed.

"After surgery, I was told to eat everything in sight to keep my weight up, and I did!"

THE PATIENT IN REMISSION

When a patient's lung cancer goes into remission, he or she can be said to be in either *"partial remission"* or *"complete remission."* Whether one is referring to a small-cell lung cancer or non-small-cell lung cancer, a partial remission is primarily said to be a "reprieve." It is a sign that the cancer has been significantly impacted by the treatment. It is also a sign that the cancer has, in general, not been eradicated. There is an exception to this rule, however. Patients with **bulky disease** in the chest receiving combined chemotherapy and radiation will frequently have a residual mass that will qualify them as being in partial, rather than complete, remission. Upwards of 15% to 20% of patients with bulky disease may in fact have no evidence of cancer in those lesions. In this case, it is appropriate to wait for a period of time and then continue with the same x-ray studies used as part of the follow-up study.

It is significant to note that a residual cancer may take many months before it resumes growing. When a patient is in a durable, **partial response** (exhibiting a favorable reaction to treatment; eg, a reduction in the size of tumor), or seems to have a complete disappearance of his or her cancer, then the initial tests used for measurement should be continued. The frequency with which these tests are performed changes, however (as noted above). If the cancer recurs, it will need to be fully "re-staged." Thereafter, a new treatment plan will be developed based on an evaluation of prior therapy and the extent of recurrence.

THE PROBLEM OF "SECOND PRIMARY" CANCERS

An increasing problem for patients with lung cancer is the development of *second primary lung cancers*. As noted earlier, smoking causes the entire airway to be exposed to the toxic effects of cigarette

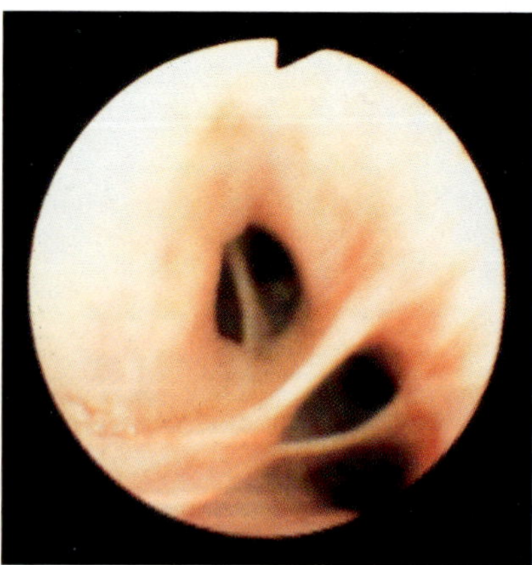

FIGURE 13A

Invisible—Bronchoscopic image of right lower lobe under white-light bronchoscopy. No abnormality was observed.

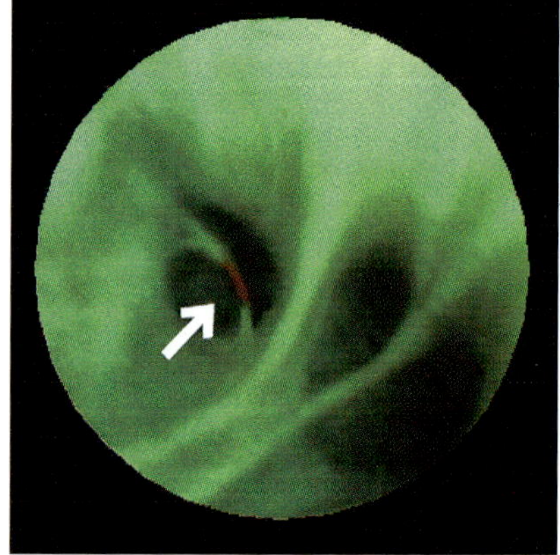

FIGURE 13B

Carcinoma in situ—Right lower lobe (same area as Figure 13A) under fluorescence bronchoscopy. A small, reddish area of abnormal fluorescence was observed near the arrow. Biopsy showed the presence of carcinoma in situ. The adjacent normal tissue fluoresced green.

smoke, and therefore, it is not unreasonable to find that other areas of the lung have also become affected in a similar fashion. Individuals cured of early stage lung cancer, or even locally advanced (regional) lung cancer, have at least a 3% per year incidence of developing a second primary cancer. Patients treated for and cured of small-cell lung cancer seem to have an even higher incidence of developing non-small-cell lung cancers. Follow-up for these individuals includes the same restaging and follow-up examinations that were performed for all previously treated lung cancer patients. However, the physician will now be interested in ways to quickly ascertain whether or not a second primary lesion has developed.

DIAGNOSIS OF A SECOND PRIMARY CANCER

The chest x-ray—obtained at least annually during follow-up treatment for lung cancer—can detect a second primary cancer. Collection of routine sputum specimens for examination of the cells under the microscope has not been a particularly effective way of evaluating patients afflicted with lung cancer. Several studies are now searching for specific molecular changes in the sputum related to lung cancer; but these are not quite ready for routine testing.

A new, promising technique called **fluorescent bronchoscopy** uses the same instrument used during the initial diagnostic bronchoscopy. This time, however, rather than just a plain white light, the light that illuminates the inside of the windpipe shines at a different fluorescent frequency. **Figures 13(A)** and **(B)** depict bronchoscopic images of both normal and abnormal findings. This light appears to be taken up differentially by cancer cells, particularly very early cancer cells, so that very early lung lesions can be identified better during this procedure than with standard bronchoscopy. This test is now routinely available in many institutions.

"I approached cancer like a full-time job. There are so many things you have to do, like getting tests and treatment. I thought, 'This is my job, and I've got to get better at it to get cured.' I did that rather than thinking about how bad it could be, and it worked. It worked."

How Can Lung Cancer Be Prevented?

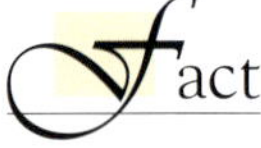

I am a heavy smoker, but if I take large doses of vitamins and antioxidants, I can prevent the development of lung cancer.

Although there are some population-wide studies suggesting that antioxidants have a beneficial effect in reducing the incidence of cancer, it has thus far been impossible to apply this to risk reduction in any individual. In reality, very little is understood about the interaction of diet in the prevention of lung cancer.

PRIMARY PREVENTION

Far and away, the simplest means of preventing cancer of the lung is to prevent individuals from ever smoking, or to convince them to stop almost immediately after they begin. This approach is called primary prevention, and unfortunately, it is the area where physicians are currently having the least success.

Adolescent Smoking: Adolescence is the traditional time for rebellion against parental dictates and "No Smoking" is one of the most frequent demands parents make. Although many adults have been convinced to stop smoking, smoking rates for adolescents, particularly young women, are rapidly rising. Most techniques used to convince adults to stop smoking are ineffective in teenagers. Various lawsuits against tobacco companies now reveal that those companies purposefully marketed their products to adolescents—It was no accident that Joe Camel was a cartoon character!

Curricular programs to prevent children from smoking result in a high degree of knowledge about the many life-threatening problems associated with smoking, but have little or no positive impact on smoking rates among teenagers. Teenagers seem to be much more influenced by peer pressure. Studies have yet to confirm the effectiveness of TV advertisements directed at adolescents' "sense of smell" and social desirability. Suffice it to say, however, that the risk of dying at 55 or 60, rather than 75 or 80, is so incredibly far in their future that smoking campaigns make little or no impact on adolescents.

Many more curricular programs aimed at early smoking cessation need to be developed. Teenagers need to nip the smoking habit in the proverbial "butt" as soon as they start. To date, however, this has been a neglected arena.

Adult Smoking: In adults, however, smoking cessation programs have been much more successful. Nicotine patches, nicotine gums, prescriptions, and various counseling programs have all shown some success in reducing adult smoking rates.

Early studies suggested that the increased risk of lung cancer does not recede for 10 to15 years after a period of significant smoking. Nevertheless, smoking cessation is vital for all adults. On the bright

TABLE 4

**CURRENT SMOKERS
INCREASED LUNG CANCER RISK***

	Men		Women	
	1-20 cig/d	>21 cig/d	1-19 cig/d	>20 cig/d
	18.8	26.9	7.3	16.3

**FORMER SMOKERS
INCREASED LUNG CANCER RISK****

	Men		Women	
	1-20 cig/d	>21 cig/d	1-19 cig/d	>20 cig/d
<1 year	26.7	50.7	7.9	34.3
1 to 2	22.4	33.2	9.1	19.5
3 to 5	16.5	20.9	2.9	14.6
6 to 10	8.7	15.0	1.0	9.1
11 to 15	6.0	12.6	N/A	N/A
>16	3.1	5.5	N/A	N/A

N/A = not available

**How to read this table:* Among current smokers, a man who smokes between 1 and 20 cigarettes per day has a risk of developing lung cancer 18.8 times greater than a man who has never smoked cigarettes. A woman who smokes between 1 and 19 cigarettes per day has a lung cancer risk 7.3 times greater than the woman who never smokes.

**A former smoker's risk of developing lung cancer is actually inecreased for up to 3 years after he or she stops smoking. Thereafter, his or her risk is reduced, and usually after 10 to 15 years of not smoking cigarettes, the former smoker's health is not significantly different from that of a lifelong non-smoker.

Source: The National Cancer Institute, 1999.

side, within 1 year of quitting, a former smoker's risk of heart disease is reduced by nearly 50% compared to someone who continues to smoke. Unfortunately, the risks for lung cancer do not rapidly decrease, but the sooner one quits smoking, the quicker one begins to benefit (**Table 4**). According to the National Cancer Institute, after 10 to 15 years of smoking cessation, most former smokers' health status is not significantly different from that of a lifelong nonsmoker. Not only does it appear to reduce the risk of developing lung cancer at a later date, but it also clearly improves the outlook for the development of severe chronic pulmonary disease, including emphysema and cardiac disease.

SECONDARY PREVENTION

Once an individual has smoked for a significant period of time (20 pack-years, give or take), he or she has significantly increased their risk of developing lung cancer. Even if he or she immediately stops smoking, given the very slow growth of these cancers, the risk will persist for many years.

Antioxidants and Natural Vitamins: Efforts to reverse the molecular, though still premalignant, changes that have occurred in the airways are known as secondary prevention. Numerous antioxidants and natural vitamins have been proposed in this regard. Studies of retinoic acid (vitamin A) have suggested a reduced incidence of cancer in those individuals who took these compounds. However, this was a very special group of patients. As explained earlier, only 10% to 15% of heavy smokers will develop lung cancer, presumably on some sort of genetic basis. Consequently, giving vitamins or antioxidants to the entire population of ex-smokers would take an enormous number of patients to decipher whether there was any difference in the development of cancer.

Individuals already cured of one lung cancer by a surgical procedure are still at increased risk of developing a second lung cancer from the impact of

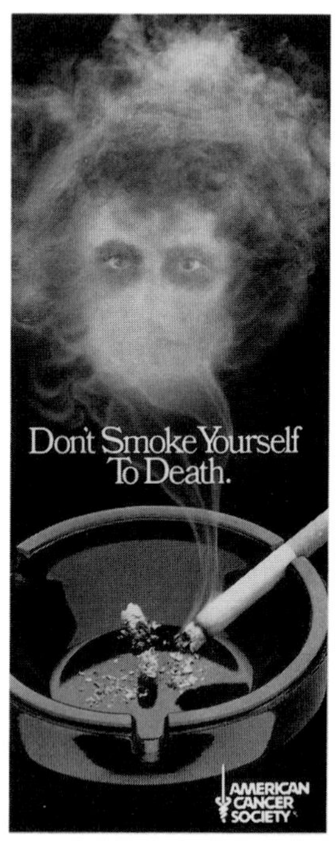

the smoke elsewhere in their airways. Several studies of the activity of vitamin A derivatives (retinol and precursor carotenes) show a reduction in this rate of second cancers. Additional large trials are presently attempting to confirm the activity of vitamin A in this situation.

Another relative of vitamin A, beta-carotene, is, however, not helpful. Two large studies in the United States and Finland have shown that smokers who took beta-carotene as part of a preventive regimen actually had an increased rate of lung cancer and a pattern of earlier death than smokers not taking beta-carotene. These studies only serve to highlight how little we know about the actual effects of these compounds on the airways.

Another antioxidant, selenium, was used in a trial to prevent the development of skin cancers. It was not successful in that respect, but it did cause a marked reduction in the number of lung cancers in that population. A study to confirm these results is just getting underway.

இ

How to Cope With Lung Cancer

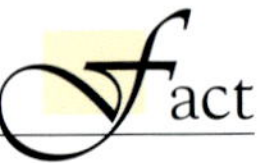

"My cancer is just going to recur and there is no way I can stop it."

In fact, your lung cancer may not recur. Even if it does, for virtually every stage of this disease, the length of time before this recurrence is now substantially longer than in the past.

Everyone with cancer fears for his or her life. Everyone with cancer fears the development of pain. Everyone with cancer fears becoming a burden on his or her family and friends. Everyone with cancer fears being unable to care for themselves and to lead a productive existence. Everyone with cancer fears treatment that goes on and on without thought to the quality of his or her existence. Everyone with cancer wants to live. Some lung cancer patients, however, bear the additional burden of guilt about having "caused" their lung cancer by smoking, despite abundant public information of its dangers. Some patients might believe they are going to die anyway from their lung cancer and may as well continue smoking. Studies have shown, however, that lung cancer patients who continue to smoke will fare much worse than those who stop smoking. Even patients who stop smoking at the time of diagnosis will have a better outlook than those who do not stop.

Additionally, some lung cancer patients suffer a profound fear that they will not be able to catch their breath and that they will smother. Many patients live with a deeply pessimistic and negative approach from family, friends, physicians, and even specialists in oncology. It's a wonder so many do so well.

SECOND OPINIONS

Dealing with cancer is a process that involves the patient and his or her entire network of family, friends, and healthcare team. Openness, a full discussion of the extent of disease, the type of envisioned treatment, and the likelihood of its success should be engaged before any therapy begins. When a patient isn't sure about his or her choices, or the utcome of these choices, and when he or she feels pushed into one form of therapy, it is time to get a second opinion. It is far better to get a second opinion before commencing therapy than when you are halfway into a course of therapy.

FAMILY INVOLVEMENT

Family members, particularly adult children, who are not present for the initial discussions about the expectations for therapy, are often the most disconnected and upset when that therapy begins to fail. The vast majority of patients and families have their own inner and familial strength that allows them to deal with the many issues related to their own or a loved one's cancer in a constructive, positive way. Our strongest possible recommendation is an open, full discussion with the entire family before therapy commences.

Fear of death becomes an issue of personal faith and is handled with varying degrees of success by most individuals and family members. Yet a very small minority of patients become so profoundly distressed that more intensive professional intervention by psychologists or psychiatrists may be required. Several mild sedatives can also reduce anxiety and fear. However, when depression or anxieties become severe, professional assistance is warranted.

DEALING WITH PAIN

Pain is a frequent unwelcome visitor to cancer, lung cancer included. There is nothing noble about trying to withstand pain. Your physician should work with you to find the best means of relieving your pain by whatever means work and are tolerable. Pain can be successfully relieved in the vast majority of patients so that they can live as normally as possible.

Weight loss can also accompany progressive cancer, or can even be a significant side effect of radiation and chemotherapy. Several medications will stimulate the appetite, and several dietary

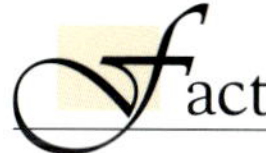

Myth

"I have no one to talk to about my lung cancer. There are so many support groups for patients with breast and prostate cancer, but hardly any for lung cancer."

Fact

There are now a growing number of support groups for lung cancer patients. Check in the back of this book for a directory of lung cancer support groups, as well as e-mail addresses, phone and fax numbers for agencies that deal specifically with lung cancer.

supplements will go a long way toward keeping your weight up. In addition, the best and most common appetite stimulant is alcohol. For those who have not had a problem with alcohol in the past, a cocktail before dinner, or a glass of wine with dinner, will often markedly improve one's appetite.

HAIR LOSS

Problems related to hair loss during chemotherapy can be dealt with several different ways. Most women will seek their own hairdresser or a special salon near their treatment facility that specializes in the care of the hair before it comes out. These places can also supply hairpieces, turbans, and other approaches to maintaining appearance. Many men will prefer to shave their entire head, rather than deal with patchy hair loss. The ever-present baseball cap seems to be the most popular approach to dealing with hair loss related to chemotherapy.

RELEASING THE GUILT

The guilt associated with having caused one's cancer by smoking is unique to lung cancer patients. Past generations of smokers could say they were unaware of the facts concerning the dangers o smoking; but it has been a couple of decades since anyone could legitimately make that claim. Again, most individuals and families are able to deal with this guilt and keep it from interfering with their day-to-day activities. Many patients and family members will go out of their way to become converts to anti-smoking campaigns and to help enlighten other family members and colleagues about the dangers of smoking. This may be particularly important for family members, who may be genetically susceptible themselves to developing cancer. I the anxiety or depression associated with this guilt gets out of hand, though, professional therapy may be required.

MANAGING BREATHING PROBLEMS

The most profound fear of lung cancer patients is the inability to breathe. In this case, maintaining contact with your primary physician, as well as your oncologist, can be of particular importance. Most individuals with lung cancer also have chronic pulmonary disease, which can be a significant source of breathing problems. Oftentimes, patients and their oncologists become wrapped up in the treatment of the lung cancer and forget about the underlying chronic pulmonary disease. Maximizing the treatment of chronic pulmonary disease with antibiotics, **bronchodilators** (medicines that open up the airways), and either inhaled or oral steroids can go a long way toward improving a patient's ability to breathe. In like manner, cardiac disease is also a common accompaniment in older individuals; appropriate treatment of heart disease will often improve breathing as well.

An accumulation of fluid around the heart or in the space between the lungs and chest wall will markedly diminish breathing capacity to the point where it can even become life threatening. Removal of the fluid and treatments to prevent its recurrence can also significantly reduce this problem.

One should never assume that a progressive loss of the capacity to breathe goes hand in hand with lung cancer. It may have a very treatable cause and should be aggressively pursued. When shortness of breath is due to a progression of the cancer, a judicious use of oxygen and intravenous morphine can significantly allay the patient's sense of breathlessness. Contrary to widespread belief, intravenous morphine is not administered in order to speed up the expected outcome for any patient with end-stage disease. Instead, morphine is used to help calm an anxious patient, to help him or her sleep better, and to also open up the airways, allowing for easier breathing and relief from the breathlessness.

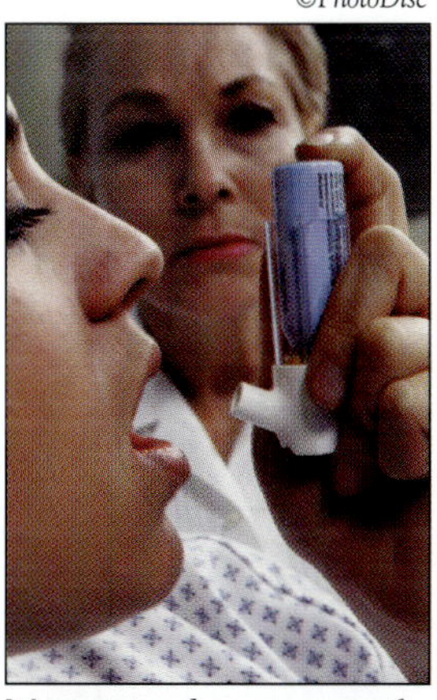

©PhotoDisc

Maximizing the treatment of chronic pulmonary disease can go a long way toward improving a patient's ability to breathe.

HOSPICES

Hospices are available in most communities to provide emotional and spiritual counseling, as well as the home-care support that may become necessary for the management of patients with end-stage lung cancer.

SUPPORT GROUPS

Most groups focused on survivorship are centered around breast and prostate cancers. There has been a shortage of support groups for lung cancer patients. This is unfortunate since lung cancer kills far more men and women than breast cancer and prostate cancer combined.

©PhotoDis

There are a growing number of support groups for lung cancer patients.

Men and women with lung cancer may feel they have no choice but to visit support groups aimed for women and men stricken with breast and prostate cancer. In these instances, these lung cancer patients will often feel that their very unique concerns are not being addressed.

There are now, however, a growing number of support groups for lung cancer patients. Most recently, a new survivor's group called the Alliance for Lung Cancer Advocacy, Support, and Education (ALCASE) has been formed by patients and family members whose loved ones did not survive the disease. This group focuses on advocacy issues for patients with lung cancer, and in particular, on increasing the amount of research support for lung cancer. ALCASE is also instrumental in establishing lung cancer support groups around the country. In some communities, the American Cancer Society is also active in providing specific support functions for lung cancer patients.

"I believe in miracles."

APPENDIX:
Support Groups and Resources for Lung Cancer Patients

Alliance for Lung Cancer Advocacy, Support, and Education (ALCASE)
1601 Lincoln Avenue
Vancouver, Washington 98660
1-(800) 298-2436
www.alcase.org

Cancer Care, Inc.
National Office
1180 Avenue of the Americas
New York, New York 10036
1-(800) 813-HOPE (4673)
www.cancercare.org
E-mail: info@cancercare.org

Cancer Information Service (CIS)
1-(800) 4-CANCER/
1-(800) 422-6237, serving all 50 states
(9:00 am - 4:30 pm) local time
Available in English and Spanish
1-(800) 332-8615 for the hearing
impaired
www.nci.nih.gov

National Coalition for Cancer Survivorship
1010 Wayne Avenue
Silver Spring, Maryland 20910
1-(888) YES-NCCS (937-6227),
9:00 am - 6:00 pm
Fax: (301) 565-9670
www.cansearch.org
E-mail: info@cansearch.org

National Hospice Organization
1901 North Moore Street, Suite 901
Arlington, Virginia 22209
(703) 243-5900
www.nho.org

PROGRAMS OFFERED BY THE AMERICAN CANCER SOCIETY

American Cancer Society (ACS)
1599 Clifton Road, NE
Atlanta, Georgia 30329
1-(404) 320-3333
National Cancer Information Center
1-(800) ACS-2345 24 hrs/7 days
www.cancer.org

CanSurmount
(1-800) ACS-2345
www.cancer.org

I Can Cope
(800) ACS-2345
www.cancer.org

Glossary

Accelerated coronary disease: A premature hardening of the coronary arteries, possibly leading to a heart attack and sudden death. Both genetically determined and avoidable risk factors, such as cigarette smoking, contribute to the disease and its earlier onset.

Adenocarcinoma: A malignant tumor made up of cancer cells that arise from the mucosa. See Bronchoalveolar carcinoma.

Adrenalin: A hormone secreted by the adrenal glands upon stimulation of the central nervous system in response to stress, anger, and/or fear, in turn, resulting in increased heart rate, blood pressure, cardiac output, and carbohydrate metabolism.

Advanced disease: See Distant disease.

Alkaline phosphatase: An enzyme produced in both the bone and liver, whose examination can be used in the clinical diagnoses of many illnesses, including lung cancer.

Alveoli: The tiny bunched air sacs located at the end of the two branches of the trachea, known as the bronchi; the site where respiration occurs.

Anaplastic lung cancers: Cancers tending to grow more rigidly and to spread earlier.

Antiemetic: An agent that prevents or alleviates nausea.

Apex: A general anatomy term used to signify the superior region of any organ or bone structure; eg, the apex of the lung extends up into the clavicle.

Apices: Plural of apex. See Apex.

Arrhythmia: Any disturbance in the heart's rhythm.

Atelectasis: An incomplete expansion, or collapse, of the lungs, as from bronchial obstruction.

Benign: Not cancerous.

Biopsy: The removal of tissue for microscopic examination in order to determine if a cancer is present.

Blood-brain barrier: A layer of tightly packed cells that make up the walls of brain capillaries and prevent many substances in the blood from entering the brain.

Bone marrow aspiration: Under local anesthesia, a needle is inserted into the marrow of the hipbone, whereupon marrow cells are aspirated and examined under a microscope.

Bone scan: A procedure where minute amounts of radioactive material are injected and a 'scan' is taken of all the body's bones to detect ongoing repair of bone due to either cancer or trauma.

Bony metastasis: The spread of a cancer to the bone.

Bronchi: The two branches of the trachea that extend into the lung; also known as the large airways.

Bronchitis: An acute or chronic inflammation of the membrane lining of the bronchial tubes; caused by infection or inhalation of irritants, such as smoke.

> **Chronic b.:** Inflammation and infection of the large airways characterized by the production of purulent (yellow or green sputum); reversible with smoking cessation and antibiotics.

Bronchoalveolar carcinomas: A variant type of adenocarcinoma of the lung; also called alveolar carcinoma, alveolar cell carcinoma, or bronchiolar carcinoma; often arises in multiple sites at the same time.

Bronchodilators: Any substance that acts to dilate constricted bronchial tubes to aid in breathing; especially used in asthma.

Bronchoscopy: A lighted, flexible, tubular instrument that is inserted into the trachea and bronchi to look for malignancy.

Bulky disease: Any cancer showing characteristics of a large tumor.

Cancer: An abnormal, uncontrolled growth of malignant cells that tend to invade surrounding tissue and spread to new body sites, such as the brain, liver, and/or bone.

Carcinoid tumor: A well-differentiated tumor arising from the hormonal cells of the lung; usually behaves benignly.

Carcinoma: An invasive, malignant tumor; synonymous with cancer.

Carcinoma in situ: A cancerous lesion contained in one area of the body; not metastasizing.

Carina: A ridge-like structure formed when the two bronchi diverge from each other.

CAT scan: A type of scan in which x-rays are used to create cross-sectional pictures of the body; also known as computerized axial tomography.

Chemotherapy: The treatment of cancer with drugs.

Chronic obstructive pulmonary disease (COPD): Any disorder marked by a persistent obstruction of bronchial airflow; eg, asthma, chronic bronchitis, and pulmonary emphysema.

Ciliated cells: Cells that are covered by minute fringes of hair, which serve to move fluid or mucous films over the surface of cells; the earliest cells damaged by smoking.

Clavicle: Either of two slender bones that extend from the sternum to the scapula; also known as the collarbone.

Cognitive dysfunction: Any disability in memory, perception, judgment, and reasoning.

Combination chemotherapy: The use of several different agents at once (usually 2 to 4) in order to enhance the effectiveness; seen particularly in cancer chemotherapy; also known as polychemotherapy.

Combined modality: The application of surgery, radiation, and chemotherapy in various combinations and sequences.

Complete remission: The shrinkage or disappearance of cancer in response to therapy so that it cannot be detected by physical exam or x-ray studies. Not synonymous with "cure," as residual microscopic disease may still exist.

Complete response: See Complete remission.

Computed tomography: See CAT scan.

Contralateral: Situated on, pertaining to, or affecting the opposite side.

Cortex: The outer region of an organ or structure.

CT scan: See CAT scan.

Dementia: Damaged brain tissue resulting in severely impaired memory and reasoning abilities.

Distant disease: A primary cancer that has spread to distant regions of the body; eg, a primary lung cancer with metastasis to the brain; also known as widespread disease.

Distant spread: See Distant disease.

Dye-contrast studies: X-rays in which a dye is given by vein so that blood vessels can be better distinguished from surrounding tissues.

Dysplasia: An abnormal development or growth of tissues, organs, or cells; cells are considered abnormal, NOT malignant.

Emphysema: A chronic disease of the lungs characterized by the destruction of the alveoli; causes irreversible loss of breathing function.

Environmental smoke: Tobacco smoke that is inhaled in any outdoor or indoor area.

Environmental exposures: Any inhaled irritant that may contribute to the development of a cancer; eg, pollution, chronic dust exposures.

Epithelium: Any tissue layer covering the body surfaces or lining the internal structures of the body cavities, tubes, and hollow organs.

Extensive small-cell lung cancer: A small-cell cancer that has spread beyond the chest; similar to the term, distant or widespread disease.

Femur: The long upper bone of the hind leg, extending from the pelvis to the knee; also known as the thighbone.

Fine-needle aspiration (FNA): A type of biopsy in which cells are removed from a lump using a needle and syringe. The cells are studied under a microscope to detect the presence of cancer cells.

Fluorescent bronchoscopy: A bronchoscopic examination, where a special fluorescent light illuminates the windpipe; useful for finding a very early cancer.

Fraction: A total dose of radiation therapy that may be divided into small doses, or fractions, and delivered over a period of time.

Gemcitabine (Gemzar): A newer nucleoside analog chemotherapy used primarily in combination therapy for non-small-cell lung cancer.

Glandular cancer: See Adenocarcinoma.

Granulomas: An inflamed, benign mass formed of granulation tissue.

Hemoptysis: Coughing up blood or bloody mucus from the lungs.

Hamartomas: A benign, tumor-like mass.

Hilar lymph nodes: Lymph nodes are the outposts of the immune system. Lymph nodes in the hilum of the lung (see below) are the first lymph nodes a lung cell will encounter. See Lymph nodes/glands.

Hilum: If one thinks of the lung as a balloon, the hilum is the "neck" of the balloon where the airway, blood vessels, nerves, etc., enter and leave the lung.

Humerus: The long upper bone of the arm, extending from the shoulder to the elbow.

Hyperfractionation: The subdivision of radiation treatment with a reduction in dose per exposure and an increase in the number of doses, but no decrease in overall treatment span; utilized in order to decrease side effects while delivering equivalent or greater anti-tumor effects.

Hyperplasia: A condition in which there is an abnormal multiplication of cells; known to be a very early premalignant change.

Intrapulmonary: Situated in the substance of the lung.

Ipsilateral: Situated on, pertaining to, or affecting the same side, as opposed to contralateral, or the other side.

Kidney toxicity: Damage to the kidneys by chemotherapy or radiation that may lead to kidney failure.

Large airways: See Bronchi.

Late intensification: Intensifying a therapy (eg, chemotherapy) after a period of standard therapy.

Lesion: Any well-defined area of disease.

Limited resection: Resections of lung portions that are smaller than a total lobe (eg, segmentectomy or wedge resection).

Limited small-cell lung cancer: Refers to a small-cell lung cancer that is confined to the chest; similar to localized or regional cancer.

Lobectomy: Each lung consists of 2 to 3 lobes that are anatomically distinct. Removal of an entire lobe (lobectomy) is the most common surgery for lung cancer.

Local disease: A condition that originates in and remains confined to one part of the body.

Local therapies: Any form of treatment (eg, radiation therapy) administered directly toward the site of disease.

Locally advanced disease: See Regional disease.

Lymph: A nearly translucent liquid composed of excess tissue fluid and proteins; fluid found in the lymphatic vessels.

Lymph nodes/glands: Small structures located throughout the body that serve as the outposts of the immune system, destroying bacteria and filtering toxic substances; connected by a system of vessels called lymphatics; can collect cancer cells that travel through the lymphatics; the presence of cancerous cells in the lymph nodes indicates that the cancer has developed the capacity to spread.

M stage: A part of the staging system used to indicate the presence of metastasis; scale ranges from M0 to M1.

Magnetic resonance imaging (MRI): A machine that produces a strong magnetic field to detail three-dimensional images of the body, regardless of intervening structures.

Malignant: Cancerous.

Malignant pleural effusion: Tumor cells involving the lining around the lungs that cause fluid to accumulate in the space between the lungs and the chest wall.

Mediastinal lymph nodes: The lymph nodes located in the mediastinal region.

Mediastinoscopy: Examination of the lymph nodes in the mediastinum by means of an endoscope; permitting direct observation and biopsy.

Mediastinum: The area in the chest that lies between the lungs; bound by the sternum, spinal column, and diaphragm; contains the esophagus, trachea, blood vessels, nerves, and lymph nodes.

Metastasis: The spread of primary cancer cells through the blood to other parts of the body; eg, the brain. When a cancer spreads to another site, it is said to have metastasized.

MRI: See Magnetic resonance imaging.

Multicentric: Arising in several sites at the same time.

Myocardial infarction: A heart attack.

N stage: A part of the staging system used to designate the extent of lymph-node involvement in lung cancer; scale ranges from N0 to N3.

Neoadjuvant therapy: Chemotherapy or radiation therapy given before surgery to help shrink a tumor.

Non-small-cell lung cancer (NSCLC): A general term comprising all lung carcinomas, except small-cell lung cancers; includes large-cell carcinoma, adenocarcinoma, bronchoalveolar carcinoma, and squamous cell cancer.

Obstructive pneumonitis: Inflammation of the lungs, causing difficult breathing.

Occupational exposures: Any exposure, such as asbestos, dust, and radon, which may instigate a cancer.

Ophthalmoscope: An instrument for viewing the interior of the eye, especially the retina; used to detect increased pressure in the brain due to metastasis to the brain.

Paclitaxel (Taxol): The original drug of the taxane family; derived from the bark of the Yew tree, but now synthetic; used in both non-small-cell and small-cell lung cancer.

Palliative care: Treatment given to relieve symptoms, not to cure disease.

Pancoast tumor: A tumor located at the top of the lung, extending outward, and destroying the ribs and vertebrae; also known as a superior sulcus tumor.

Papilledema: A swelling of the optic nerve in the back of the eye; due to increased intracranial pressure and usually signifying brain metastasis.

Parietal pleura: The membranes that cover the lungs.

Partial remission: A partial diminishment or shrinkage of cancer; residual cancer is still present, however. Most clinicians require a 50% shrinkage to label a response "partial."

Partial response: See Partial remission.

Performance status: A measure that clinicians use to evaluate a patient's well being and to help determine whether he or she will be able to tolerate chemotherapy.

Pericardial effusion: Inflammation of the sac that surrounds the heart; associated with an accumulation of fluid (pericardial fluid) that interferes with the heart's ability to pump. May be due to infection, cancer, or a side effect of some treatments.

Peripheral vascular disease: Disease affecting the blood vessels.

Pleura: The lining around the inside of the chest.

Pleural effusion: The presence of excess (pleural) fluid in the space between the lungs and chest wall.

Pneumonia: Infection of the lungs themselves. Characterized by fever, cough, and production of purulent (yellow or green) sputum.

Pneumonectomy: The surgical excision of an entire lung in an effort to remove a cancerous tumor(s).

Polychemotherapy: See Combination chemotherapy.

Primary malignancies: See Primary tumor.

Primary tumor: The site of origin of any carcinoma; also known as primary cancers, primary carcinomas, and primary malignancies.

Prophylactic cranial irradiation: Radiation given to help prevent lung cancer spread to the brain.

Prophylactic therapies: Treatment administered to help prevent development of secondary cancers or metastases.

Purulent: Containing pus.

Radiation therapy: Treatment of disease with radiation by means of x-rays, ionizing radiation, and ingestion of radioisotopes.

Recurrence: A reappearance of a cancer. There are three kinds of recurrences: local—at the original site; regional—near the original site; or distant—at another site of the body; eg, brain.

Refractory: See Resistant.

Regional disease: Any cancer that is limited to or affecting a certain region of the body; eg, the chest area.

Resistant: Not readily yielding to treatment; also known as refractory.

Response: A reaction to treatment.

> **Complete response:** No evidence of disease following treatment.
>
> **Partial response:** A limited reduction in tumor size noted in response to treatment.
>
> **No response:** The absence of any discernable favorable reaction to treatment or, in fact, worsening of the disease.

Secondary cancer: A cancer that has spread from its point of origin to another site in the body.

Second primary lung cancers: The development of a new lung cancer after treatment of a prior lung cancer.

Secretory zone: A central zone of the lung.

Sleeve resection: A surgical procedure to remove a portion of the lung or lung tissue.

Small-cell lung cancer (SCLC): A common, highly malignant form of lung carcinoma arising from the hormonal cells of the lung.

Smoker's cough: A cough instigated by the toxic effects of cigarette smoke.

Spiculated: Needle-like.

Spinal cord: The main "electrical" cord extending from the brain down through the spinal canal and encased in the spine itself. Numerous branches or roots extend from the spine to allow sensation and movement of all body parts.

Spirometry: A test to measure lung and/or breathing capacity.

Spontaneous cancers: Any cancer occurring without an external influence.

Squamous cancer: One of the three types of non-small-cell lung cancers originating from the squamous epithelium.

Staging: The process of determining all characteristics of any cancer by taking specific tests then assigning varying levels of the T stage (tumor size), N stage (nodal status), M stage (presence of metastasis), then Stages 1 through 4. See T stage, N stage, and M stage.

Superior sulcus tumor: See Pancoast tumor.

Superior vena cava: The upper portions of either of the two large veins that discharge blood into the right atrium of the heart.

Supraclavicular lymph nodes: The lymph nodes located just above the clavicle, or collarbone.

Swallowing tube: See Esophagus.

Synergistic effect: An interaction of elements whose combined effect is greater than the sum of its parts.

T stage: A measurement scale denoting the size of the tumor and whether the tumor involves adjacent vital structures; stages generally range from T1 through T4.

Topotecan (Hycamtin): A newer drug that interferes with DNA replication; used primarily in small-cell lung cancer.

Trachea: The tube that extends from the larynx to the bronchi; the chief passageway of air to and from the lungs; also known as the windpipe.

Tumor: The abnormal growth of cells that can be either benign or malignant.

Tumor markers: A biochemical substance found, for instance, in the blood, which indicates a biologic activity or presence of cancer; eg, CEA (carcinoembryonic antigen); used to screen, diagnose, assess prognosis, follow response to treatment, and monitor for recurrence; not always specific for cancer and not often used in the management of lung cancer.

Vinorelbine (Navelbine): A newer drug of the vinca alkaloids; derived from mistletoe; used primarily for non-small-cell lung cancer.

Widespread disease: See Distant disease.

Windpipe: See Trachea.

X-ray: A type of radiation. Low doses of x-rays are used to diagnose disease; high doses of x-rays are used to treat cancer. The term "x-ray" is frequently used to refer to the picture created with x-rays.